Surgical Management of Facial Trauma

Editors

KOFI DEREK O. BOAHENE
ANTHONY E. BRISSETT

OTOLARYNGOLOGIC CLINICS OF NORTH AMERICA

www.oto.theclinics.com

October 2013 • Volume 46 • Number 5

ELSEVIER

1600 John F. Kennedy Boulevard • Suite 1800 • Philadelphia, Pennsylvania, 19103-2899

http://www.oto.theclinics.com

OTOLARYNGOLOGIC CLINICS OF NORTH AMERICA Volume 46, Number 5
October 2013 ISSN 0030-6665, ISBN-13: 978-0-323-22731-5

Editor: Joanne Husovski
Development Editor: Donald Mumford

Otolaryngologic Clinics of North America (ISSN 0030-6665) is published bimonthly by Elsevier, Inc., 360 Park Avenue South, New York, NY 10010-1710. Months of issue are February, April, June, August, October, and December. Business and Editorial Offices: 1600 John F. Kennedy Blvd., Suite 1800, Philadelphia, PA 19103-2899. Customer Service Office: 6277 Sea Harbor Drive, Orlando, FL 32887-4800. Periodicals postage paid at New York, NY and additional mailing offices. Subscription prices are $348.00 per year (US individuals), $653.00 per year (US institutions), $167.00 per year (US student/resident), $460.00 per year (Canadian individuals), $819.00 per year (Canadian institutions), $516.00 per year (international individuals), $819.00 per year (international institutions), $258.00 per year (international & Canadian student/resident). Foreign air speed delivery is included in all *Clinics'* subscription prices. All prices are subject to change without notice. **POSTMASTER:** Send address changes to *Otolaryngologic Clinics of North America*, Elsevier Health Sciences Division, Subscription Customer Service, 3251 Riverport Lane, Maryland Heights, MO 63043. **Telephone: 1-800-654-2452 (U.S. and Canada); 314-447-8871 (outside U.S. and Canada). Fax: 314-447-8029. E-mail: journalscustomerservice-usa@elsevier.com (for print support); journalsonlinesupport-usa@elsevier.com (for online support).**

Reprints. For copies of 100 or more of articles in this publication, please contact the Commercial Reprints Department, Elsevier Inc., 360 Park Avenue South, New York, NY 10010-1710. Tel.: 212-633-3874; Fax: 212-633-3820; E-mail: reprints@elsevier.com.

Otolaryngologic Clinics of North America is also published in Spanish by McGraw-Hill Interamericana Editores S.A., P.O. Box 5-237, 06500 Mexico D.F., Mexico.

Otolaryngologic Clinics of North America is covered in *MEDLINE/PubMed (Index Medicus), Current Contents/Clinical Medicine, Excerpta Medica, BIOSIS, Science Citation Index,* and *ISI/BIOMED.*

Printed and bound by CPI Group (UK) Ltd, Croydon, CR0 4YY

Transferred to digital print 2012

Contributors

EDITORS

KOFI DEREK O. BOAHENE, MD, FACS
Associate Professor, Department of Otolaryngology Head and Neck Surgery, The Johns Hopkins School of Medicine, Baltimore, Maryland

ANTHONY E. BRISSETT, MD
Director of Facial Plastic and Reconstructive Surgery, Bobby R. Alford Department of Otolaryngology - Head and Neck Surgery, Baylor College of Medicine, Facial Plastic Surgery Center, Houston, Texas

AUTHORS

DANIEL S. ALAM, MD
Head, Section of Facial Plastic & Reconstructive Surgery, Head & Neck Institute, Cleveland Clinic Foundation; Associate Professor of Surgery, Lerner School of Medicine, Case Western Reserve University, Cleveland, Ohio

FARHAD ARDESHIRPOUR, MD
Department of Otolaryngology, Head and Neck Surgery, University of Minnesota, Minneapolis, Minnesota

KOFI DEREK O. BOAHENE, MD, FACS
Associate Professor, Department of Otolaryngology Head and Neck Surgery, The Johns Hopkins School of Medicine, Baltimore, Maryland

ANTHONY E. BRISSETT, MD
Director of Facial Plastic and Reconstructive Surgery, Bobby R. Alford Department of Otolaryngology - Head and Neck Surgery, Baylor College of Medicine, Facial Plastic Surgery Center, Houston, Texas

RYAN BROWN, MD
Assistant Professor, Department of Head and Neck Surgery; Staff Surgeon, Kaiser Permanente, Denver, Colorado

PATRICK J. BYRNE, MD
Director, Division of Facial Plastic and Reconstructive Surgery, Johns Hopkins School of Medicine, Baltimore, Maryland

JOHN J. CHI, MD
Assistant Professor, Division of Facial Plastic & Reconstructive Surgery, Washington University School of Medicine, St Louis, Missouri

YADRANKO DUCIC, MD, FRCS(C), FACS
Clinical Professor, Department of Otolaryngology–Head and Neck Surgery, University of Texas Southwestern Medical Center, Dallas; Otolaryngology and Facial Plastic Surgery Associates, Fort Worth, Texas

MICHAEL A. FRITZ, MD, FACS
Department of Otolaryngology—Head and Neck Surgery, Head and Neck Institute,
Cleveland Clinic Foundation, Cleveland, Ohio

JOSEPH N. GIACOMETTI, MD
Fellow, Department of Ophthalmology, Cullen Eye Institute, Baylor College of Medicine,
Houston, Texas

AUSTIN GRAY, DDS
Department of Otolaryngology, Greater Baltimore Medical Center, Baltimore, Maryland

W. MARSHALL GUY, MD
Bobby R. Alford Department of Otolaryngology-Head and Neck Surgery, Baylor College
of Medicine, Houston, Texas

TIMOTHY M. HAFFEY, MD
Department of Otolaryngology—Head and Neck Surgery, Head and Neck Institute,
Cleveland Clinic Foundation, Cleveland, Ohio

PETER A. HILGER, MD
Department of Otolaryngology, Head and Neck Surgery, University of Minnesota,
Minneapolis, Minnesota

LARRY H. HOLLIER Jr, MD, FACS
Division of Plastic Surgery, Michael E. Debakey Department of Surgery, Baylor College of
Medicine, Houston, Texas

DAVID Y. KHECHOYAN, MD
Division of Plastic Surgery, Michael E. Debakey Department of Surgery, Baylor College of
Medicine, Houston, Texas

AMIT KOCHHAR, MD
Department of Otolaryngology, Head and Neck Surgery, Johns Hopkins School of
Medicine, Baltimore, Maryland

LINDA N. LEE, MD
Fellow, Facial Plastic and Reconstructive Surgery; Department of Otolaryngology Head
and Neck Surgery, The Johns Hopkins School of Medicine, Baltimore, Maryland

SEONGMU LEE, MD
Private Practice, Sylmar, Los Angeles, California

ALICE C. LIN, MD
Division of Head and Neck Oncology, Massachusetts Eye and Ear infirmary,
Massachusetts General Hospital, Harvard Medical School, Boston, Massachusetts

DERRICK T. LIN, MD
Co-Director of the MGH/MEEI Cranial Base Center, Division of Head and Neck Oncology,
Massachusetts Eye and Ear infirmary, Massachusetts General Hospital, Harvard Medical
School, Boston, Massachusetts

SOFIA LYFORD-PIKE, MD
Chief Resident, Department of Otolaryngology Head and Neck Surgery, The Johns
Hopkins School of Medicine, Baltimore, Maryland

RALPH MAGRITZ, MD
Consultant, Department of Oto-Rhino-Laryngology, Head and Neck Surgery,
Prosper-Hospital, Academic Teaching Hospital, Ruhr University Bochum, Recklinghausen,
Germany

LAURA A. MONSON, MD
Division of Plastic Surgery, Michael E. Debakey Department of Surgery, Baylor College of
Medicine, Houston, Texas

CHRISTOPHER R. OLYNIK, DMD, FRCD(C)
Department of Otolaryngology, Greater Baltimore Medical Center, Baltimore, Maryland

RAJA SAWHNEY, MD, MFA
Assistant Professor, Department of Otolaryngology–Head and Neck Surgery, University
of Florida, Gainesville, Florida

DAVID A. SHAYE, MD
Department of Otolaryngology, Head and Neck Surgery, University of Minnesota,
Minneapolis, Minnesota

RALF SIEGERT, MD, DDS, PhD
Director, Department of Oto-Rhino-Laryngology, Head and Neck Surgery,
Prosper-Hospital, Academic Teaching Hospital, Ruhr University Bochum, Recklinghausen,
Germany

GHASSAN G. SINADA, DDS
Maxillofacial Prosthodontist, Department of Otolaryngology, Greater Baltimore Medical
Center, Baltimore, Maryland

E. BRADLEY STRONG, MD
Professor, Department of Otolaryngology-Head and Neck Surgery, University of
California Davis Medical Center, Sacramento, California

TRAVIS T. TOLLEFSON, MD, MPH
Associate Professor, Department of Otolaryngology-Head and Neck Surgery, University
of California Davis Medical Center, Sacramento, California

WILLIAM M. WEATHERS, MD
Division of Plastic Surgery, Michael E. Debakey Department of Surgery, Baylor College of
Medicine, Houston, Texas

JOHN O. WIRTHLIN, DDS, MSD
Division of Plastic Surgery, Michael E. Debakey Department of Surgery, Baylor College of
Medicine, Houston, Texas

ERIK M. WOLFSWINKEL, BS
Division of Plastic Surgery, Michael E. Debakey Department of Surgery, Baylor College of
Medicine, Houston, Texas

MICHAEL T. YEN, MD
Associate Professor, Department of Ophthalmology, Cullen Eye Institute, Baylor College
of Medicine, Houston, Texas

Contents

reattachment technique. A satisfactory primary reconstruction is not always possible to obtain and the remaining defects must be reconstructed secondary. The localization of the defect, its extent, and the condition of the tissue surrounding the defect are essential criteria for further treatment planning. This article provides an overview of the treatment of acute auricular trauma and of important aspects of secondary defect repair of the pinna.

Surgical Management of Facial Trauma

OTOLARYNGOLOGIC CLINICS OF NORTH AMERICA

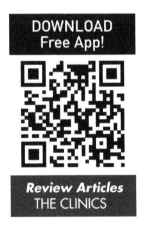

**DOWNLOAD
Free App!**

Review Articles
THE CLINICS

NOW AVAILABLE FOR YOUR iPhone and iPad

Preface

Contemporary Management of Facial Trauma

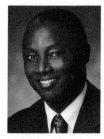 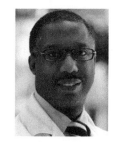

Kofi Derek O. Boahene, MD   Anthony E. Brissett, MD, FACS
Editors

The principles for managing maxillofacial trauma are well established. However, the rapid evolution of technology has broadened the options available in evaluating, planning, and repairing these injuries. In this edition, we address the contemporary management of skeletal and soft tissue injuries within the head and neck following trauma. To provide a broad view, authors from multiple subspecialty disciplines were invited to contribute their experience. In this issue, the authors have been given the latitude to structure their information in an unconstrained style in order to pass on their expertise in an unhindered manner.

There is extensive coverage of dentoalveolar injuries, rarely seen in most trauma textbooks. The article on auricular trauma provides in-depth coverage of ear reconstruction from simple local flap repair to complicated microvascular transfer of prefabricated costochondrial ear constructs. In the past, patients with traumatic auricular avulsion who failed reimplantation were offered prosthetic reconstruction as their only option. The result of prefabricated ear reconstruction described here shows that autologous tissue repair can provide results comparable to that of prosthetic ears. Worldwide, over 24 face transplants have been successfully performed, mostly for extensive traumatic injuries. With the increasing success of face transplants, composite tissue allografts have technically become a viable option for treating massive craniofacial injuries. A number of patients who have undergone face transplantation had failed multiple autologous free tissue transfer. The indications and outcomes for the vascularized transfer of composite tissue autograft and allograft for massive traumatic facial injuries are extensively covered in this text. In addition, we offer a

Otolaryngol Clin N Am 46 (2013) xi–xii
http://dx.doi.org/10.1016/j.otc.2013.09.002
0030-6665/13/$ – see front matter © 2013 Published by Elsevier Inc.

oto.theclinics.com

comprehensive discussion highlighting the contemporary management of classically described traumatic injuries.

We are grateful to all the authors who have shared their extensive expertise.

Kofi Derek O. Boahene, MD
Department of Otolaryngology - Head and Neck Surgery
Johns Hopkins Facial Plastic and Reconstructive Surgery Center
Baltimore, MD, USA

Anthony E. Brissett, MD, FACS
Director of Facial Plastic and Reconstructive Surgery
Bobby R. Alford Department of Otolaryngology - Head and Neck Surgery
Baylor College of Medicine
Facial Plastic Surgery Center
Houston, TX, USA

E-mail addresses:
dboahen1@jhmi.edu (K.D.O. Boahene)
brissett@bcm.edu (A.E. Brissett)

Radiology in Facial Trauma

Intraoperative Use of CT Imaging

E. Bradley Strong, MD*, Travis T. Tollefson, MD, MPH

KEYWORDS

- Computed tomography • Intraoperative imaging • Maxillofacial trauma
- Cone beam CT • Fan beam CT • Intraoperative CT • Facial fracture

KEY POINTS

- Intraoperative computed tomography likely has a role in complex congenital, traumatic, and/or oncologic facial deformities.
- There is low level support for this hypothesis in the literature.
- Although many surgeons think intraoperative imaging is beneficial in complex cases, high-quality prospective outcomes research will be required to determine the appropriate indications for the use of intraoperative computed tomography.

INTRODUCTION

In 1895 Wilhelm Rontgen discovered electron beam radiation and coined the term "x-ray." In 1903 William Coolidge developed the x-ray tube, which was further refined and is in clinical use today. Plain radiographs are the fundamental tools used for diagnosis and treatment of long bone fractures. Preoperative radiographs are used for diagnosis and treatment. Intraoperative and postoperative radiographs are routinely obtained to assure adequate reduction and appropriate implant positioning.

Before the advent of computed tomography (CT), plain radiographs were also the modality of choice for the diagnosis and treatment planning of maxillofacial injuries. However, intraoperative and postoperative radiographs were not routinely used. Studies evaluating the efficacy of postoperative plain radiographs have not found them to be beneficial,[1–4] most likely due to the limited resolution of plain radiographs in determining the accuracy of fracture reduction and implant placement, as well as the potential risk associated with radiation exposure to the vital structures of the head and neck.

The development of CT is credited to Godfrey Hounsfield and Allan Cormack in 1972. The specificity, sensitivity, and resolution of CT in midfacial fractures is

Funding and Disclosures: None.
Department of Otolaryngology-Head and Neck Surgery, University of California Davis Medical Center, 2521 Stockton Boulevard, Suite 7200, Sacramento, CA 95817, USA
* Corresponding author.
E-mail address: edward.strong@ucdmc.ucdavis.edu

significantly greater than plain radiographs[5,6] and greater than or equal to that of panorex images for the mandible.[7] Since its clinical introduction, CT has revolutionized head and neck diagnostic imaging and has become the gold standard for diagnosis and treatment planning of maxillofacial injuries.

With the increased availability of CT in the 1990s, some surgeons began to use CT for postoperative confirmation of fracture reduction and implant positioning. The more recent addition of portable scanners has brought the question of intraoperative imaging to the forefront. The few studies, which have looked at the efficacy of intraoperative CT scans for maxillofacial trauma, have been supportive of the technique.[8-11] However the question of efficacy remains unanswered. Is intraoperative and postoperative CT imaging beneficial for maxillofacial reconstructive surgery? Although currently there are no answers to this question, this article reviews the current literature, discusses the different CT modalities that are available, and presents the authors' clinical experience with the use of intraoperative CT for maxillofacial trauma and reconstruction.

TECHNOLOGY

X-ray CT can be divided into 2 different modalities, computed axial tomography (CAT) and digital volume tomography (DVT). Computed axial tomography scanners are also called "fan beam" scanners because of the "fan" shape of the x-ray photons that are emitted. These scanners are composed of an x-ray tube, a collimator to shape the beam, and a series of detector arrays opposite to the x-ray tube, all contained within a circular gantry. As the patient passes though the gantry, the x-ray tube moves in a circle around the patient. The x-ray beam is variably absorbed by the tissues, and the density differences are then recorded by a sensor array (**Fig. 1**). Information is then presented as a series of axial slices: one slice per sensor. Current CT scanners typically obtain between 64 and 256 slices per rotation. DVT scanners are also called "cone beam" scanners because of the "cone" shape of the x-ray photons that are emitted. Unlike fan beam scanners, there is no collimator, only a source and a sensor.

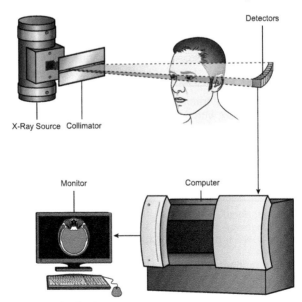

Fig. 1. The components of a fan beam CT scanner.

The sensor is a generally a "flat panel" screen that records the pattern of tissue absorption (**Fig. 2**). There is no collimator; therefore, the tissue density differences are recorded as a *volume* of data that can be sliced in any dimension without significant image degradation (**Fig. 3**). Subsequent descriptions in this article use the terms "fan beam CT" and "cone beam DVT" to reference these 2 different technologies. The term "CT" will be used to describe the general modality of x-ray CT.

Radiation Dose

The effective radiation doses associated with traditional fan beam CT scans of the maxillofacial region are low, ranging from 600 to 800 microsieverts. Some comparative numbers include background radiation, 8 microsieverts (24 h); lateral cephalogram, 6 microsieverts; dental series, 171 microsieverts. However, recent studies have brought into question the long-term risk of radiation exposure related to CT scans.[12,13] Although cone beam DVT generates less patient dosage (40–80 microseiverts) than fan beam CT,[14] a comparison between the 2 techniques raises some complex issues. First, there is no universally accepted common dose metric to compare the 2 techniques. Also, direct comparison of the modalities is complicated by the lack of equivalent image quality (particularly soft tissue resolution).[15] Finally, because cone beam DVT systems usually operate with an automated exposure system, control of patient dosage can be more difficult than with fan beam CT.[16]

Contrast Resolution/Image Quality

The image quality and contrast resolution of traditional fan beam CT is superior to cone beam DVT because the cone beam DVT does not have a collimator (resulting in greater x-ray scatter) and the characteristic of the flat panel detector.[17] However, cone beam DVT provides near equivalent bony resolution (**Fig. 4**).

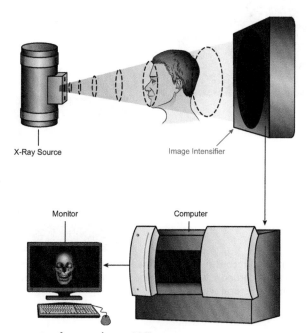

X-Ray Source   Image Intensifier

Monitor   Computer

Fig. 2. The components of a cone beam DVT scanner.

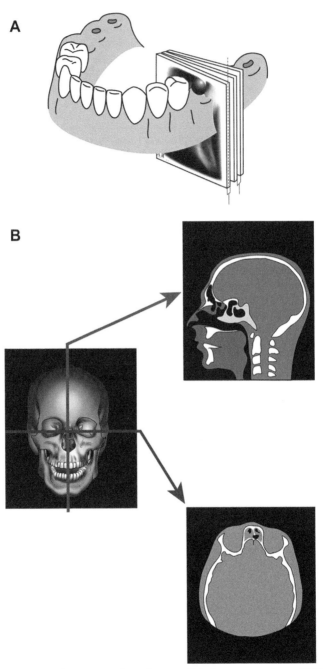

Fig. 3. Three-dimensional reconstruction of a mandible from a cone beam DVT scanner (*A*). Note that the data are recorded as a 3-dimensional volume, but can be sliced in any plane to obtain 2-dimensional structural representations (*B*).

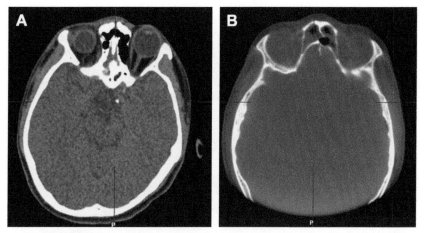

Fig. 4. (A) An axial slice of a head CT taken from a fan beam CT scanner. Note the soft tissues of the brain and orbit are demarcated. (B) An axial slice of a head CT taken from a cone beam DVT scanner. Note that the soft tissues of the brain and orbit are poorly defined. However bone resolution is similar.

Configuration and Portability

Fan beam CT scanners have a circular "closed gantry" structure, which the patient passes through. There are stationary, in hospital scanners, and portable configurations (**Fig. 5**). Cone beam DVT scanners vary in configuration, but typically have an open gantry format that looks very similar to a c-arm (**Fig. 6**). There are also hybrid

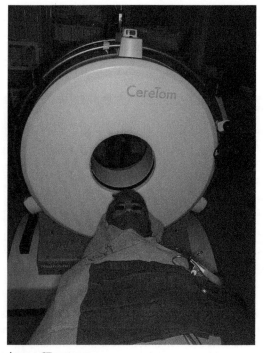

Fig. 5. Portable fan beam CT scanner.

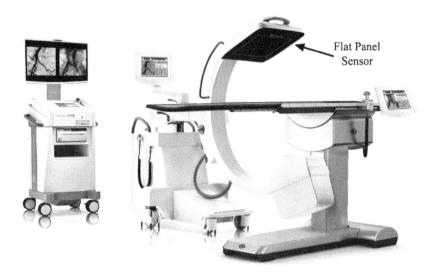

Fig. 6. Physical configuration of an open gantry fan beam DVT scanner with a flat panel sensor. (*Courtesy of* Ziehm Imaging, Inc, Nuremberg, Germany; with permission.)

configurations that are open to position the patient and closed to scan (**Fig. 7**). Stationary cone beam DVT scanners exist (ex. interventional angiography), but they are beyond the scope of this article.

Field of View

Fan beam CT scanners typically obtain data as the patient moves through the gantry on a motorized bed, allowing an essentially "unlimited" field of view along the length of the patient. In contrast, cone beam DVT scanners are stationary in the axial dimension and rotate around the patient to collect data. Because there is no longitudinal motion

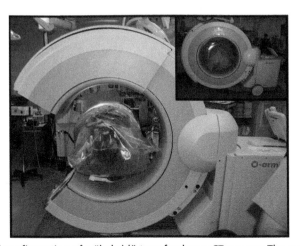

Fig. 7. Physical configuration of a "hybrid"-type fan beam CT scanner. The gantry is open to position the patient and closed to scan (inset). Note the c-arm drape (central image) that is passed over the patient and bed to maintain patient sterility.

along the axis of the patient, the longitudinal field of view is limited by the width of the flat panel sensor (see **Fig. 6**). Current flat panel sensors range in size from 12 to 40 cm in width. A width greater than approximately 25 cm will allow imaging of the entire skull with one scan.

Gantry Size

Stationary, in-hospital fan beam CT scanners have a gantry diameter of approximately 70 to 75 cm, allowing access to the vast majority of patients. The rotation diameter of the c-arm type cone beam DVT scanners is similar (see **Fig. 6**), allowing scans of the head and neck as well as body. However some closed gantry scanners, with smaller patient opening size, only allow access for the patient's head. Because the shoulders cannot be accommodated within the gantry, imaging of the mandible is limited or impossible (see **Fig. 5**).

INDICATIONS

The clinical indications for intraoperative CT scanning are poorly defined and largely based on surgeon preference. Factors that may influence the decision to use intraoperative CT include access to the equipment, fracture location and severity, concerns about radiation exposure, as well as a limited number of studies evaluating the efficacy of this technique.

Access

Not all institutions have access to portable CT scanners. Typical costs range from $200,000 to $850,000. The authors have found that an effective strategy for purchase of a portable CT system is to generate support from multiple services, commonly including neurosurgery and pediatric surgery. Both have critically ill patients in the intensive care unit. Transport of such patients may entail significant risk related to dislocation of access lines (ie, intravenous, ventilators, extracorporeal membrane oxygenation devices). The use of portable CT scanners in the intensive care unit has been shown to reduce the risk of adverse events related to transport. In addition, the cost-effectiveness of introducing portable CT scanners at the Cleveland Clinic was suggested to provide a return on investment in as early as 7 months after inception.[18] The orthopedic and neurosurgical spine services may also benefit from the use of intraoperative CT.

Fracture Location and Severity

The most effective treatment for fractures that can be well visualized is adequate exposure and accurate alignment of the bony segments. Thus there is no indication for intraoperative imaging. Some examples include noncomminuted fractures of the anterior mandible, minimally displaced and noncomminuted zygoma fractures, simple orbital floor/medial wall fractures, frontal sinus fractures treated with an open technique, and alveolar ridge fractures. More complex injuries in which all fracture lines are not be well visualized can be considered for intraoperative imaging. These more complex injuries include complex mandible and zygoma fractures with marked rotation or comminution; complex orbital fractures; naso-orbito-ethmoid fractures; and complex skull base reconstructions.

Radiation Exposure

Although it is possible to estimate levels of radiation exposure for any given device, the long-term consequences to the patient are difficult to quantify. The current literature has been able to correlate some association between the effective doses of radiation from

CT scans with some degree of increased risk (ie, malignancy, cataract), particularly in the pediatric population.[12,13] Therefore, when using intraoperative CT, the surgeon must perform a risk-benefit analysis for which both the potential risk and the benefit remain ill defined. The authors have attempted to limit intraoperative scanning to adult patients with complex reconstructive needs related to trauma or tumor extirpation. A secondary intraoperative dilemma is faced after a scan is obtained, and the initial repair is inadequate. Once the reduction is revised, the surgeon must decide whether to perform a final scan to document the reduction or avoid a second scan and assume the reduction was adequate. The authors have not typically repeated a scan.

Literature

In 1999 Stanley[8] was one of the first surgeons to study intraoperative CT for maxillofacial trauma. He evaluated 25 patients undergoing surgical treatment of unilateral zygoma and/or orbital blowout fractures. Intraoperatively, major revisions were performed in 2 patients and minor revisions were performed in 5 patients. The author concluded that it was a viable technique that could reduce the incidence of bony malreduction at the time of acute repair rather than during costly and more difficult delayed revisions. He also hypothesized that for selected cases, intraoperative CT may eliminate the need for direct visualization of all fracture sites while still ensuring an adequate reduction.

In 2001 Hoelzle and colleagues[9] evaluated 29 patients with orbito-zygomatic fractures (12 orbital and 17 orbito-zygomatic) using intraoperative, postreduction CT scans. Three of the orbito-zygomatic fractures were repaired with a closed reduction. None of these required a revision. Of the 26 remaining cases, 4 (15%) underwent an intraoperative revision as indicated by the CT (1 isolated orbit and 4 orbito-zygomatic fractures). These findings suggest that minimally displaced orbito-zygomatic fractures, not requiring open reduction, are less likely to need intraoperative imaging, whereas more complex fractures may benefit from the technique.

In 2011 Rabie and colleagues[10] did a feasibility study looking at intraoperative cone beam CT evaluation of facial fractures using the Xoran xCAT scanner (Xoran Technologies, Inc, Ann Arbor, MI, USA). The study included only 3 patients: a multiply comminuted anterior/posterior table frontal sinus fracture, and 2 complex maxillomandibular "pan facial" fractures. The authors reported 2 of the 3 patients required in intraoperative revision after a scan was obtained. One patient required a revision of the frontal sinus cranialization and one patient required an open repair of a subcondylar fracture that was found to be malreduced after a closed reduction.

Later in 2011 Ibrahim and colleagues[11] studied the utility of intraoperative CT as both a clinical and a teaching tool for facial fracture repair. Resident physicians (PGY 4–8) were allowed to expose and reduce facial fractures. The reduction was then evaluated by an attending physician and an intraoperative CT was obtained. The authors reported that 3 of the 7 fractures (43%) required an acute revision at the time of surgery. They concluded that fractures that involve both the horizontal and the vertical facial buttresses on multiple levels were the most likely to require an intraoperative revision.

INTRAOPERATIVE SCAN TECHNIQUE

The development of an efficient intraoperative CT scanning protocol requires coordination between the surgeon, the operating room staff, and the department of radiology. This coordination will assure that the room is properly configured and that the scanner is available at the appropriate time.

Room Setup

Portable CT scanners have a relatively large footprint, ranging from approximately 0.75 × 1.30 m to 1.0 × 2.75 m. The surgeon and staff must take this into consideration when setting up the room. The authors have found the most efficient technique is to have the patient's head rotated 180° away from anesthesia and lined up toward the side of the room with the operating room door. Consideration must be given to the location of electrical cords and other equipment, such as headlights, instrument tables, and navigation systems, which will all need to be moved before scanning the patient.

Patient Preparation

Preoperative planning for the bed configuration and patient positioning is critical. Some scanners require a radiolucent head holder that must be attached to the bed before the patient is placed on the operating table. These head holders are often narrow and may require extra padding to avoid pressure points around the neck and shoulders.

Patient Sterility

Intraoperative sterility can be maintained by draping either the CT scanner or patient. Although most portable CT scanners have sterile covers that can be purchased, the authors have found them to be cumbersome. An effective alternative is to simply place a c-arm drape over the entire head of the bed and patient (see **Fig. 7**). This drape maintains patient sterility while allowing the CT technician to make minor adjustments in patient position before scanning.

Time

Coordination with the department of radiology can drastically reduce the time necessary for acquisition of an intraoperative CT scan. To reduce the risk of time wasted in transport or unexpected technical difficulties with the scanner, the authors generally contact the department of radiology the morning of surgery with an estimate of the hour that the scanner will be required. Approximately 30 to 45 minutes before the scanner is needed, the CT technician is contacted and the scanner is transported to a location directly outside the room. Even if the operating room is large enough to accommodate the scanner before use, it is kept outside the room until just before it is used. The authors have found that the device limits mobility and generates a significant amount of background noise that can be undesirable. Once the surgical reconstruction is accomplished, all equipment surrounding the head of the bed is moved aside, and the scanner is brought into the room and positioned at the head of the bed. The surgeon is concurrently covering the patient with a c-arm drape. The technician can then position the scanner over the patient without concerns about sterility. Nonessential personnel leave the room while the scan is obtained. The actual scan time generally takes less than 1 minute. Finally, the surgeon can evaluate the reduction in 3 planes to determine the adequacy of the repair. On average, the entire process, from bringing the scanner into the room to reading the scan, takes between 10 and 20 minutes. The room preparation and the experience of the CT technician have been found to be the most important factors in reducing the overall time required to obtain the scan.

ADJUNCTIVE TECHNIQUES: INTRAOPERATIVE NAVIGATION

Repair of complex congenital, traumatic, or oncologic facial deformities can be extremely challenging. Presurgical virtual planning combined with intraoperative navigation, rapid prototype models, and drill or cutting guides can be beneficial. Because intraoperative navigation does not result in added radiation exposure to the patient, it can be used in a much more dynamic way. The surgeon may reduce a bone segment or place dynamic mesh and rapidly get feedback about position and contour. If unsatisfied, the surgeon can reposition the bone or implant and immediately evaluate the modification. When the surgeon feels that the positioning has been optimized, an intraoperative CT is performed for final confirmation. In the authors' experience, this technique improves the intraoperative accuracy and reduces the risk of an inadequate repair when the final intraoperative CT is obtained.

CLINICAL CASE

The patient was a 21-year-old man involved in a motor vehicle accident who presented early in the authors' experience of using intraoperative CT. The patient sustained a left orbito-zygomatic fracture. Physical examination revealed mild diplopia in upward gaze without gross entrapment, moderate flattening of the left malar eminence, and normal sensation over the V_2 nerve distribution (**Fig. 8**). Preoperative CT revealed a noncomminuted, moderately displaced left orbito-zygomatic fracture (**Fig. 9**). The patient was taken to the operating room and the fracture was exposed with left sublabial and transconjunctival incisions. The zygoma was reduced with some effort. The inferior orbital rim and floor seemed to be well reduced. However, despite significant effort, the zygomatico-maxillary buttress reduction was thought

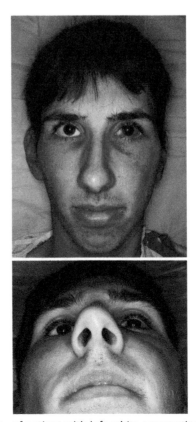

Fig. 8. Preoperative photo of patient with left orbito-zygomatic fracture.

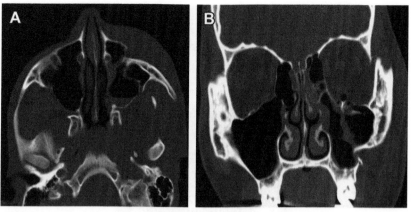

Fig. 9. Preoperative axial (*A*) and coronal (*B*) fan beam CT scan of left orbito-zygomatic fracture.

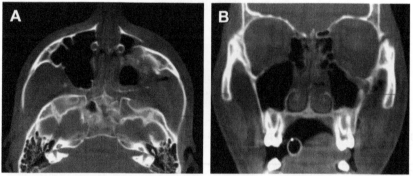

Fig. 10. Intraoperative axial (*A*) and coronal (*B*) cone beam DVT scan revealing an adequate orbital reduction, but inadequate reduction of the zygomatico-maxillary buttress.

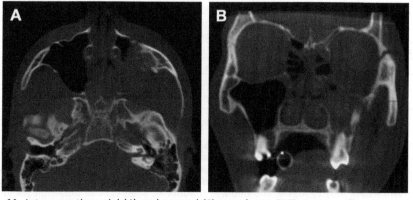

Fig. 11. Intraoperative axial (*A*) and coronal (*B*) cone beam DVT scan revealing a complete fracture reduction.

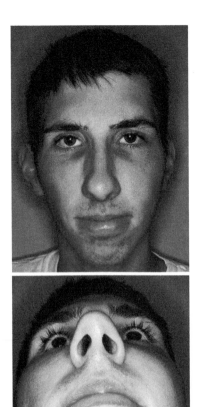

Fig. 12. Postoperative photo of patient status after left orbito-zygomatic fracture reduction.

Table 1 Summary: intraoperative CT	
	Example
Advantages	
Minimize surgical exposure	Reduce the subperiosteal dissection necessary to visually verify the fracture reduction
Reduce incidence of revision procedures	Inadequate fracture reduction can be identified with intraoperative CT and corrected in same setting
Disadvantages	
Time	20 min OR time[a]
Cost	$200,000–$850,000[b]
Radiation exposure	40–800 microSieverts[c]

[a] Timing and coordination with technician and nurses are necessary to reduce excessive wait times for scan capture.
[b] Possible cost sharing with other services (orthopedics, neurosurgery).
[c] Additional cumulative radiation exposure, but would be comparable with a postoperative CT.[14,15]

Data from Hirota S, Nakao N, Yamamoto S, et al. Cone-beam CT with flat-panel-detector digital angiography system: early experience in abdominal interventional procedures. Cardiovasc Intervent Radiol 2006;29:1034–8; and Gupta R, Grasruck M, Suess C, et al. Ultra-high resolution flat-panel volume CT: fundamental principles, design architecture, and system characterization. Eur Radiol 2006;16:1191–205.

to be in question. Intraoperative CT was performed revealing appropriate reduction of the orbital fracture component but malreduction of the zygomatico-maxillary buttress (**Fig. 10**). A more aggressive dissection was performed with greater skeletonization over the malar eminence and zygomatic root. A more accurate reduction was eventually thought to be achieved. Although this is not the authors' current protocol, a second intraoperative CT was obtained revealing an accurate reduction (**Fig. 11**). Postoperatively the patient had an uneventful recovery with adequate symmetry and the return of normal extraocular muscle function (**Fig. 12**).

SUMMARY

Intraoperative CT likely has a role in complex congenital, traumatic, and/or oncologic facial deformities (**Table 1**). There is a low level of support for this hypothesis in the literature. Although many surgeons think the intraoperative imaging is beneficial in complex cases, high-quality prospective outcomes research is required to determine the appropriate indications for the use of intraoperative CT.

REFERENCES

1. Jain MK, Alexander M. The need of postoperative radiographs in maxillofacial fractures—a prospective multicentric study. Br J Oral Maxillofac Surg 2009;47: 525–9.
2. Crighton LA, Koppel DA. The value of postoperative radiographs in the management of zygomatic fractures: prospective study. Br J Oral Maxillofac Surg 2007; 45:51–3.
3. van den Bergh B, Goey Y, Forouzanfar T. Postoperative radiographs after maxillofacial trauma: sense or nonsense? Int J Oral Maxillofac Surg 2011;40:1373–6.
4. Bali N, Lopes V. An audit of the effectiveness of postoperative radiographs—do they make a difference? Br J Oral Maxillofac Surg 2004;42:331–4.
5. Tanrikulu R, Erol B. Comparison of computed tomography with conventional radiography for midfacial fractures. Dentomaxillofac Radiol 2001;30:141–6.
6. Laine FJ, Conway WF, Laskin DM. Radiology of maxillofacial trauma. Curr Probl Diagn Radiol 1993;22:145–88.
7. Roth FS, Kokoska MS, Awwad EE, et al. The identification of mandible fractures by helical computed tomography and panorex tomography. J Craniofac Surg 2005;16:394–9.
8. Stanley RB. Use of intraoperative computed tomography during repair of orbitozygomatic fractures. Arch Facial Plast Surg 1999;1:19–24.
9. Hoelzle F, Klein M, Schwerdtner O, et al. Intraoperative computed tomography with the mobile CT Tomoscan M during surgical treatment of orbital fractures. Int J Oral Maxillofac Surg 2001;30:26–31.
10. Rabie AN, Ibrahim AM, Lee BT, et al. Use of intraoperative computed tomography in complex facial fracture reduction and fixation. J Craniofac Surg 2011;22: 1466–7.
11. Ibrahim AM, Rabie AN, Lee BT, et al. Intraoperative CT: a teaching tool for the management of complex facial fracture fixation in surgical training. J Surg Educ 2011;68:437–41.
12. Brenner DJ, Hall EJ. Computed tomography: an increasing source of radiation exposure. N Engl J Med 2007;357(22):2277–84.
13. Thrall J. Radiation exposure in ct scanning and risk: where are we? Radiology 2012;264:325–8.

14. Hirota S, Nakao N, Yamamoto S, et al. Cone-beam CT with flat-panel-detector digital angiography system: early experience in abdominal interventional procedures. Cardiovasc Intervent Radiol 2006;29:1034–8.

15. Gupta R, Grasruck M, Suess C, et al. Ultra-high resolution flat-panel volume CT: fundamental principles, design architecture, and system characterization. Eur Radiol 2006;16:1191–205.

16. Orth RC, Wallace MJ, Kuo MD. C-arm cone-beam CT: general principles and technical considerations for use in interventional radiology. J Vasc Interv Radiol 2008;19:814–21.

17. Miracle AC, Mukherji SK. Conebeam CT of the head and neck, part 1: physical principles. AJNR Am J Neuroradiol 2009;30(6):1088–95.

18. Masaryk T, Kolonick R, Painter T, et al. The economic and clinical benefits of portable head/neck CT imaging in the intensive care unit. Radiol Manage 2008; 30(2):50–4.

Skeletal Facial Trauma

Contemporary Management of Traumatic Fractures of the Frontal Sinus

W. Marshall Guy, MD[a], Anthony E. Brissett, MD[b],*

KEYWORDS

- Frontal sinus fracture • Frontal sinus trauma • Cranialization
- Frontal sinus obliteration • Mucocele • Frontal sinus drill out

KEY POINTS

- Frontal sinus fractures require a significant amount of force and often present with concomitant intracranial injuries.
- Appropriate initial management helps to prevent complications including infections, cerebrospinal fluid leak, and mucocele formation.
- Management strategies for frontal sinus fractures involve the prevention of early and late complications.
- Minimally invasive approaches and endoscopic techniques are increasingly being used for the effective management of frontal sinus fractures.

 Video demonstration of a frontal sinus drill-out accompanies this article at http://www.oto.theclinics.com/

INTRODUCTION

The frontal sinus is the last of the paranasal sinuses to develop, and takes on a triangular or trapezoidal shape (**Fig. 1**). Although the functions of the paranasal sinus are not fully understood, theories include lightening the skull and cushioning the brain from blunt forces and traumatic injuries by dispersing incoming forces. The frontal sinus is generally a bilateral structure, but may be unilateral in up to 15% of patients and may be absent in 8% of the population.[1] Lying anteriorly is the frontal table, posteriorly is the posterior table separating the brain from the sinus, and inferiorly is the orbital roof and frontal sinus outflow tract (**Fig. 2**).[2] The frontal sinus outflow tract is limited

[a] Bobby R. Alford Department of Otolaryngology-Head and Neck Surgery, Baylor College of Medicine, 6501 Fannin Suite NA 102, Houston, Texas 77030, USA; [b] Bobby R. Alford Department of Otolaryngology-Head and Neck Surgery, Baylor Facial Plastic Surgery Center, Smith Tower Suite 1701 6550 Fannin Street Houston, Texas 77030, USA
* Corresponding author.
E-mail address: brissett@bcm.edu

Otolaryngol Clin N Am 46 (2013) 733–748
http://dx.doi.org/10.1016/j.otc.2013.07.005
0030-6665/13/$ – see front matter © 2013 Elsevier Inc. All rights reserved.

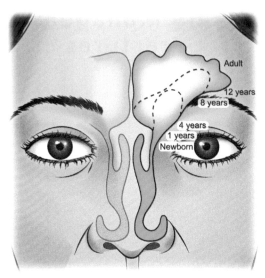

Fig. 1. Development of the frontal sinus based on age as it takes on its adult size and shape.

anteriorly by the frontal process of the maxilla forming the frontal beak. The medial wall of the outflow tract is the olfactory fossa, and the lateral wall is formed by the lamina papyracea separating the orbit from the sinus. The posterior limit is the bulla ethmoidalis, the roof being formed by the fovea ethmoidalis with the anterior ethmoidal artery coursing across it.[3]

The frontal bones and the resultant frontal sinuses represent one of the strongest structures in the face.[4] As a result, a significant amount of force is required to fracture them in comparison with other structures of the head and neck (**Table 1**).[5] Frontal sinus fractures are thus frequently associated with multiple concomitant injuries, including intracranial injuries. Frontal sinus fractures account for 5% to 15% of all

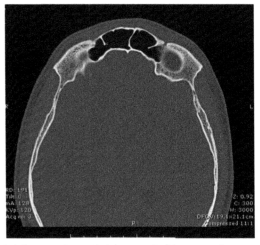

Fig. 2. Normal frontal sinus anatomy. Axial computed tomography scan of the frontal sinus showing well-aerated frontal sinus with the intersinus septum.

Table 1
Force required to fracture the facial bones

Location	Force Required for Fracture (lb)
Mandible	425–925
Maxilla	140–445
Zygoma	208–475
Frontal bones	800–2200
Nasal bones	25–75

1 lb = 0.45 kg. Note the greater force required to fracture the frontal bones in comparison with the other bones.

facial fractures[6] and are associated with various high-velocity and low-velocity causes such as motor vehicle accidents, gunshots, falls, and assaults.[7]

Injuries to the frontal sinus can be categorized into fractures that involve the anterior table, the posterior table, the outflow tract, or a combination of the 3; they can be further described as nondisplaced, displaced, or comminuted (**Fig. 3**).

ASSESSMENT AND DIAGNOSIS

The primary goal when treating frontal sinus fractures depends on the type and severity of the fracture. Cosmetic outcomes and the correction of contour irregularities are a high priority when considering the treatment goals of isolated anterior table fractures.[2] If the posterior table is involved, the primary treatment goal is to separate the intracranial contents from the sinus, minimizing the potential for intracranial complications such as cerebrospinal fluid (CSF) leaks, sinusitis, and intracranial infections. When fractures of the frontal sinus involve the outflow tract or nasal frontal recess, it is imperative to take into account the potential for long-term or late complications such as locally destructive or infectious lesions (eg, mucoceles and mucopyoceles).

PREOPERATIVE PLANNING AND PREPARATION

A high index of suspicion for frontal sinus injuries is required for all patients presenting with trauma to the upper face. Signs and symptoms that may represent a fracture of the frontal bones and the paranasal sinuses include swelling of the soft tissues,

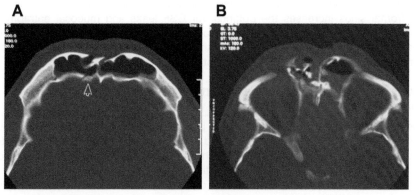

Fig. 3. Frontal sinus fractures. The *arrow* is pointing to a posterior table fracture. Anterior and posterior table frontal sinus fracture (*A*) and frontal outflow tract fracture (*B*).

contour irregularities that become more prominent as the edema resolves, hypesthesia in the first trigeminal nerve distribution, anosmia from shearing of the adjacent cribriform plate, and intracranial injuries.[4] More extensive injuries involving both the anterior and posterior table may have leakage of CSF or exposed intracranial contents.[4] Sensation to the forehead is supplied by branches of the first division of the trigeminal nerve through both the supraorbital and supratrochlear nerves; for this reason, sensation should be documented before operative repair. In addition, the frontal branch of the facial nerve courses from lateral to medial in the upper face, and may be damaged with significant lacerations of the upper face. The integrity of this branch should be evaluated and its function documented.[4]

Despite the importance of documenting the physical examination findings, radiographic imaging is the gold standard for diagnosis and classifying fractures of the frontal sinus. To properly assess the fracture, a computed tomography (CT) scan with fine cuts should be obtained. Reconstruction of the images in coronal and sagittal orientations further aids in surgical planning, particularly when assessing the frontal sinus outflow tracts.

TREATMENT GOALS FOR FRONTAL SINUS FRACTURES

The primary goal when treating frontal sinus fractures is to prevent the formation of early and late complications while attempting to restore form and function. Early complications have been described as problems that occur with the first 6 months of the injury and include, but are not limited to, sinusitis and meningitis. Late complications, on the other hand, can occur decades after the original traumatic event and may include findings such as bone erosion, mucoceles, mucopyoceles, and brain abscesses.

Although the perceived goals of treatment for frontal sinus injuries have remained relatively constant over the years, the specifics related to intervention and surgical treatments have evolved. For example, traditional philosophies emphasized either obliteration or cranialization when considering the management of frontal sinus fractures involving the frontal recess or outflow tracts.[8–10] By contrast, current literature leans toward a more conservative approach when treating fractures of the frontal recess, with preservation of form and function.[11]

Debate also surrounds the treatment algorithms when considering fractures of the posterior table. While most will agree that large comminuted fractures of the posterior table are often best treated with cranialization or obliteration, the treatment options for mild to moderately displaced posterior table fractures have a spectrum. Tightly adherent dura combined with deep mucosal invaginations on the posterior table of the frontal sinus increases the potential for CSF leaks and mucosal entrapment, respectively. For this reason, some argue for an obliterative procedure in the presence of any posterior table fracture,[8] whereas others will only intervene in the presence of a persistent CSF leak or if there is significant displacement.

PROCEDURAL APPROACH TO SINUS FRACTURES
Anterior Table Fractures

The goal for treating anterior table fractures is to restore form and improve appearance. The degree of displacement is approximated by visual and palpable contour irregularities and is confirmed by radiologic imaging. When determining the severity of the contour irregularity it is important to allow the soft-tissue swelling to resolve; this process may take 7 to 10 days depending on the nature of the trauma and the severity of the injury.

For fractures that are minimally displaced and have only a slight contour irregularity, injectable fillers such as calcium hydroxyapatite or poly-L-lactic acid can be applied.

For more significantly displaced anterior table fractures with moderate contour irregularities, the option of an overlay camouflage graft or open reduction with internal fixation (ORIF) may be exercised (**Fig. 4**). Camouflage grafts with porous polyethylene and/or titanium mesh can be placed with a minimally invasive endoscopic technique or an open approach.

Fractures and contour irregularities can be visualized from a multitude of approaches such as pretrichial, upper eyelid, or supra-brow. If a laceration is present, this too can be used to visualize the fracture. When using the endoscopic approach, 2 to 3 vertical incisions approximately 1 cm in length are made just behind the hairline. The positioning of the incisions will depend on the location and sidedness of the fracture. The incision is taken down to the subperiosteal plane and an optical cavity is elevated over the forehead to the level of the brow, being sure to avoid damage to the supratrochlear and supraorbital neurovascular bundles. Once the fracture is exposed, a small external incision can be made within a relaxed skin-tension line overlying the fracture site, allowing for placement of a bone hook to assist in elevating and reducing the depressed segment. In addition, an implant can be deployed from any of the endoscopy access ports and secured with screws through small external incisions within the relaxed skin-tension lines of the forehead.[12,13]

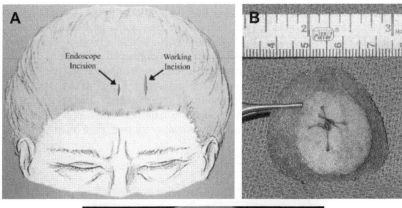

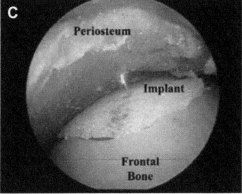

Fig. 4. Endoscopic approach to the frontal sinus. (*A*) Proposed incisions for the endoscopic approach. (*B*) Size of the implant. (*C*) Endoscopic deployment of the implant. (*A; From* Strong EB. Endoscopic repair of anterior table frontal sinus fractures. Facial Plast Surg 2009;25(1):43–8; with permission.)

For severely displaced or comminuted fractures of the anterior table, open access to the bony fragments is often necessary. Depending on the severity and location of the fracture and characteristics of the patient such as rhytids, hairline, and expectations, a variety of external approaches are available, which include using the laceration, if available; a butterfly or "open-sky" incision placed above the brow, the direct approach whereby the incision is placed within a rhytid; a pretrichial incision; or a hemicoronal or coronal approach (**Fig. 5**).

The butterfly approach uses an incision that is placed just above the eyebrow and extends medially into the glabella, connecting to an identical incision on the contralateral side. Although this approach provides good exposure to low and medially located anterior table fractures, this open-sky incision leaves a visible scar and also places the supraorbital and supratrochlear neurovascular bundles at risk, resulting in hypesthesia in the V1 distribution. The direct approach involves placing an incision in a prominent forehead rhytid directly over the fracture or using an existing laceration, but this approach suffers from the same limitations as the butterfly incision.[4] Despite their limitations, the direct or open-skin approach may provide the best access and outcome when treating patients who are bald, have a high hairline, or have a history of hair loss.

A novel technique for treating isolated anterior table fractures involves placing the incision into the tarsal crease of the upper eyelid. The orbicularis oculi and frontalis muscles are divided, and a periosteal incision is made along the supraorbital rim. A 5-mm burr is used to create a small window in the supraorbital bone, allowing an instrument to be inserted along the underside of the fracture to raise the depressed fragment. An endoscope can be used to confirm reduction.[14]

Depending on the location and extent of the fracture, a hemicoronal or coronal incision may be the best option, as this approach provides the greatest access to the entirety of the frontal sinus. The incision is made approximately 2 cm posterior to the hairline. The incision is taken down through the galea and dissection is completed in a subgaleal plane. As the supraorbital ridge is approached, care must be exercised

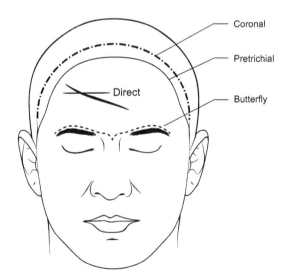

Fig. 5. Various surgical approaches to the frontal sinus, including through an existing laceration (*crosswise line*), butterfly or open-sky incision (*dotted lines*), direct approach (*dashed lines*), pretrichial approach (*solid line*), and coronal approach (*dot-dash line*).

to avoid damage to the frontal branch of the facial nerve as well the supraorbital and supratrochlear neurovascular bundles.[2,4] Although the hemicoronal or coronal incision provides outstanding access to fractures involving the frontal sinus, it is associated with hypesthesia, facial nerve weakness, and alopecia.

Once the fracture is exposed, further treatment depends on the extent of injuries. When treating isolated anterior table fractures, the fragments or segments should be identified, reduced, and fixated. In general, the reduced fragments can be stabilized with either miniplates or microplates. When bone fragments larger than 1 cm are missing, an autogenous bone graft such as calvaria, or alloplastic implants such as a titanium mesh plate or porous polyethylene, can be used to span the defect and prevent contour irregularities.[4]

Posterior Table Fractures

The management of posterior table fractures has evolved over the past decade. Concomitant injuries often dictate the treatment options, as can the presence of acute complications such as a CSF leak. Treatment options for posterior table fractures include observation, ORIF, obliteration of the frontal sinus, or removal of the posterior table with cranialization.

To maximize exposure, posterior table fractures are best approached through a coronal incision with the concomitant creation of an extended pericranial flap. In addition, posterior table fractures are rarely isolated and are typically associated with anterior table fractures. With this in mind, the fractured portions of the anterior table will need to be identified, removed, and preserved for replating. If the full extent of the frontal sinus needs to be exposed for evaluation and treatment of the posterior table, this can be accomplished with a multitude of techniques. Traditionally the use of a 6-foot Caldwell film has been used to map the shape and size of the frontal sinus. This method, however, is often imprecise, and newer more accurate options for mapping the frontal sinus are available. For example, the boundaries of the frontal sinus can be easily established with transillumination from the nasal frontal recess or through a frontal sinus trephine using nasal endoscopes (**Fig. 6**). In addition, image guidance can be used to help determine the limits of the frontal sinus and prevent inadvertent entry into the intracranial compartment. Once defined, a reciprocating

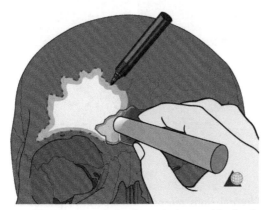

Fig. 6. Endoscopic transillumination of the frontal sinus, with the frontal sinus borders being outlined. (*Courtesy of* AO Foundation, Davos, Switzerland. AO Surgery Reference. Available at: https://www.aofoundation.org/wps/portal/surgery.)

saw or a cutting burr on a drill can be used to trace the outlined sinus. Recently the authors have begun using the piezoelectric saw to cut through the bone of the anterior table. A benefit over traditional cutting instruments includes the lack of macrovibrations, which allows for better control and helps to minimize the risk of adjacent soft tissue accidentally being brought into the saw. Once the perimeter of the frontal sinus has been osteotomized, the intersinus septum can be released with the use of a curved osteotome, allowing for removal of the remaining anterior table and exposure of the posterior table fracture.

If obliteration or cranialization of the posterior table fracture is going to be performed, the sinus mucosa of the posterior table and nasal frontal recess should be grossly removed, and the area should be drilled and polished under loupe or microscopic magnification to ensure removal of the mucosa within the invaginations of the posterior table (**Fig. 7**). After verifying that the posterior table dura is intact and there is no CSF leak, the frontal sinus cavity may be obliterated; this can be done by plugging the outflow tract with harvested temporalis muscle and a tissue sealant. The cavity itself can be obliterated by using fat harvested from the abdomen or the previously elevated pericranial flap. In addition, other materials have been proposed for obliteration, including methyl methacrylate, hydroxyapatite, allogenic lyophilized cartilage chips,[15] spontaneous frontal sinus osteogenesis,[16] and demineralized bone matrix.[17]

For fractures that involve more than 25% of the posterior table, cranialization should be considered. The process of cranialization is believed to decrease the potential of CSF leaks by directly examining and repairing the dura if needed. In addition, by removing the remaining posterior table including the mucosa and bone, one is less likely to develop long-term complications such as mucoceles and mucopyoceles. Fragments of the posterior table can be removed with the piezoelectric saw or

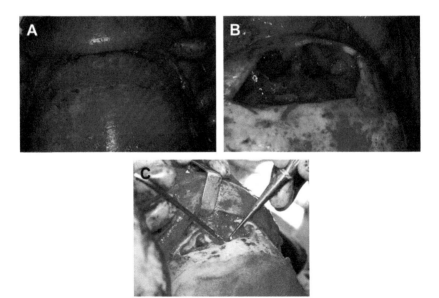

Fig. 7. Removal of frontal sinus mucosa. Intraoperative photos showing elevation of the coronal flap with visualization of the fractured anterior table (*A*), the frontal sinus mucosa visualized following elevation of the osteoplastic flap (*B*), and drilling of the mucosa (*C*).

backbiting instruments to prevent damage to the underlying dura. If any dural tears are encountered they should be repaired, and a neurosurgery consultation should be considered to assist with closure. The previously elevated pericranial flap can also be considered for dural repair if needed. Following removal of the posterior table and obstruction of the outflow ducts, the bone of the anterior table is replaced and secured in place using titanium plating systems.[2,4]

Frontal Recess Injuries

Isolated injuries of the frontal recess are uncommon. More commonly, injuries of the frontal recess are associated with concomitant injuries of the anterior table, posterior table, or naso-orbital ethmoid complex. Traditionally, reparative strategies for injuries of the frontal sinus that involved nasal frontal recess injuries would include destruction of the duct and cranialization or obliteration of the sinus. More contemporary management of frontal sinus fractures have taken a conservative approach, with the focus being preservation of form and function.

Endoscopic approaches

The endonasal/endoscopic approach to frontal recess fractures is designed to open the outflow tract, and is described as a modified endoscopic Lothrop procedure or a Draf type III procedure. The use of endoscopic navigational equipment is essential when performing this procedure, given the close proximity of the anterior cranial fossa and orbits. The nasal cavity is prepared using a topical anesthetic and decongestant, either topical 4% cocaine or 1% lidocaine with epinephrine 1:100,000 injection, with topical oxymetazoline-soaked pledgets. The axilla above the middle turbinate is injected with a lidocaine/epinephrine solution to assist with hemostasis. A powered microdebrider is used to denude the mucosa above the middle turbinate up to the nasal roof as well as the adjacent septal mucosa. The bone and cartilage is removed to create a septal window for improved instrumentation. A cutting burr is used to drill the maxillary bone to the overlying skin connecting the frontal sinus to the nasal cavity. If needed, the process is repeated on the contralateral side. Once both floors are exposed, the intersinus septum is taken down using an angled cutting burr near the superior aspect of the sinus to avoid damage to the skull base near the cribriform plate. The openings can then be widened anteriorly and inferiorly, again avoiding damage to the skull base (**Fig. 8**, Video 1).[3]

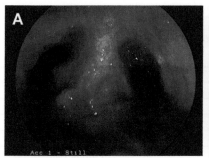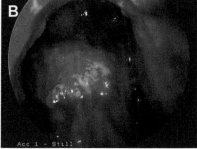

Fig. 8. Intraoperative endoscopic approach to the frontal sinus drill-out, with the frontal outflow tracts visualized (*A*) and the frontal sinus drill-out complete (*B*). (*Courtesy of* Masayoshi Takashima, MD, Houston, Texas.)

COMPLICATIONS

The primary treatment goal of most facial injuries is to preserve both form and function. By contrast, treatment of the frontal sinus is unique in that the primary goal is to prevent early and late complications, with the preservation of form and function being a secondary consideration in the treatment algorithm. Complications of frontal sinus fractures can be divided into early or late (**Table 2**). Early complications occur within the first 6 months of the injury and typically include sinusitis, hematoma, wound infection, CSF leaks, and meningitis. Late complications can occur any time after 6 months and include CSF leaks, hypesthesia, persistent contour irregularities, meningitis, mucoceles, mucopyoceles, brain abscesses, and chronic pain (**Fig. 9**).[18] Retrospective studies have reported long-term complication rates of 10% for those undergoing intervention, with 6% developing meningitis, 6% developing a mucocele, and 1% developing chronic frontal pain. It is noteworthy that these complications were found to develop as many as 25 years after the original incident.[19] Against this background it is essential that patients with frontal sinus fractures be informed about the signs and symptoms related to complications of frontal sinus fractures, and the possibility of a long-term delay in their presentation. It is also important that the physician treating these patients sustains long-term follow-up.

Cerebrospinal Fluid Leak

Determining the presence of a CSF leak is important when deciding on appropriate treatment options. Verification of a CSF leak can be performed by sending a sample for β2-transferrin analysis.[20] However, if the frontal sinus outflow tract is obstructed, there may be no rhinorrhea but only radiographic evidence of persistent sinus opacification.[15] Once verified, a trial of diversion of CSF to evaluate for spontaneous closure may be attempted, which is best accomplished with a continuous lumbar drain. If the leak persists despite conservative management, more aggressive treatment with identification and repair of the dura followed by possible cranialization or obliteration should be considered.[21,22] Of note, studies have shown up to a 10-fold increase in the risk of meningitis if a CSF fistula remains present for more than 7 days,[23] underscoring the importance of early intervention if a CSF leak is suspected.

Sinusitis/Meningitis/Infection

The frontal sinus drains naturally through venules known as the foramina of Breschet (**Fig. 10**) into the dural veins, allowing for an easy intracranial spread of infection. Debate surrounds the use of prophylactic antibiotics, with a large meta-analysis failing

Table 2	
Early and late complications of frontal sinus fractures based on time course	
Early (Within 6 mo)	**Late (After 6 mo)**
Sinusitis	Cosmetic deformity
Meningitis	Mucocele
Hematoma	Mucopyocele
Wound infection	Brain abscess
Cerebrospinal fluid leak	Hypesthesia
	Chronic pain
	Cerebrospinal fluid leak
	Meningitis

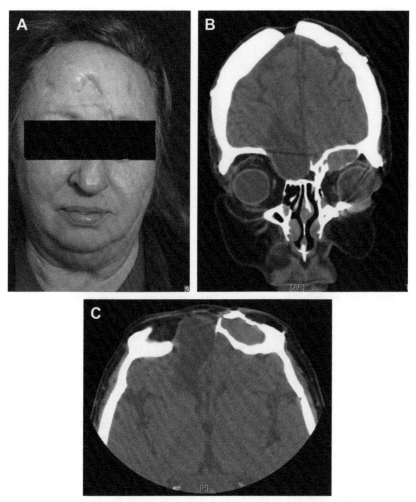

Fig. 9. Complications of frontal sinus fractures. (*A*) A contour irregularity with bony erosion of a patient with a frontal sinus fracture repaired with cranialization. Not visible is that the left eye is pushed down and out from a mucocele. (*B*) Coronal computed tomography scan of the same patient showing the encephalocele over the right eye and the mucocele pushing the left eye down and out. (*C*) Axial computed tomography scan of the same patient showing complete erosion of the anterior and posterior tables.

to show a significant decrease in the risk of meningitis.[24] These data must also be weighed against the risk of developing opportunistic infections and selecting for resistant flora. If meningitis does develop it should be managed with the assistance of an infectious disease specialist, and its cause needs to be determined. If there is a persistent CSF leak or mucopyocele, this too should be addressed.

Mucocele

Mucocele formation can occur when there is obstruction of the frontal sinus outflow tract or via the mechanical obstruction of mucosal glands.[25] Treatment involves addressing the cause of the mucocele and draining the mucocele. Endoscopic

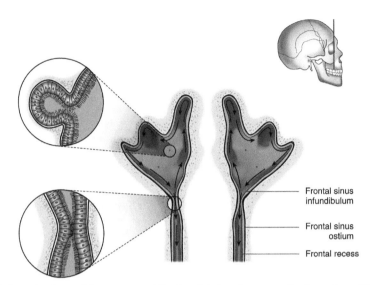

Frontal sinus
infundibulum

Frontal sinus
ostium

Frontal recess

Fig. 10. Invaginations of the mucosa of the frontal sinus known as the foramina of Breschet. These areas must be drilled to prevent the late complication of a mucocele.

management has been demonstrated to be effective at addressing frontal sinus mucoceles using either a Draf IIa, IIb, or III procedure, with restenosis of the outflow tract being most common after a Draf IIb procedure.[26] Open approaches such as obliteration or cranialization have been shown to be effective in treating the problem, although recurrence rates have been reported to be as high as 25%.[27]

Cosmetic Deformity

Patients with frontal sinus fractures may have any number of cosmetic consequences, given the high force required for the fracture. Scars that may develop in the area of the injury as a result of traumatic lacerations can be revised and refined secondarily. Patients may also identify concern with contour irregularities in the area of repair. For subtle contour irregularities, hydroxyapatite cement or other injectable fillers have been shown to be effective in providing a smoother surface.[28]

Although the plates used for repair are generally thin, patients may complain of palpable plates and request their removal. Removal of these plates can be safely performed after 6 months of the initial repair if necessary.

POSTPROCEDURAL CARE

Standard postoperative care is performed on patients with external incisions. Patients should avoid any increased pressure in the nasal cavity that could disrupt any anastomosis or place air into the soft tissue or intracranial area. Patients should be placed on stool softeners and encouraged not to enact a Valsalva maneuver. Nasal saline irrigations should be done in the immediate postoperative period to help maintain patency of the frontal sinus duct for those patients in whom the frontal sinus function has been preserved.

OUTCOMES OF SINUS FRACTURE

Given the variety of injuries that can be sustained with a frontal sinus fracture, the outcomes can vary from no residual complications or cosmetic deformities to intracranial

Clinical results in the literature		
Study	**N**	**Results**
Rodriguez et al,[10] 2008	857	Observation of frontal sinus fracture is acceptable if there is no obstructed outflow tract (3.1% complication rate)
		Fat obliteration has a 22% complication rate
		Osteoneogenesis has a 42.9% complication rate
		Cranialization has a 10% complication rate
Pollock et al,[9] 2012	154	Observation performed in 38%
		Cranialization performed in 35% with a 6% complication rate
Choi et al,[29] 2012	875	68 posterior table fractures; 9 died of original injuries
		78% managed nonoperatively
		2% complication rate (intracranial infection)
Tedaldi et al,[30] 2010	112	All patients treated surgically
		12.5% complication rate
		2.7% CSF rhinorrhea
		2.7% persistent temporoparietal headaches
		1.8% scar retraction
		5.4% limited range of extraocular motility
Chen et al,[31] 2006	78	Group 1: Observation (NFOT)
		Group 2: ORIF anterior table with sinus preservation, no involvement of the NFOT
		Group 3: ORIF anterior table, sinus obliteration, involvement of the NFOT
		Group 4: Cranialization when the posterior table was involved
		16.7% complication rate
		7.7% CSF leak
		1.3% meningitis
		5.1% wound infection
		1.3% frontal sinusitis
		1.3% frontal mucopyocele
Lakhani et al,[32] 2001	12	Group 1: Isolated anterior table fractures repaired using bony fragments attached to titanium mesh
		Group 2: Anterior table fracture with NFOT involvement repaired with sinus obliteration and anterior wall reconstruction with bony fragments attached to mesh
		Group 3: Anterior and posterior table fracture treated with cranialization and anterior wall reconstruction with bony fragments attached to titanium mesh
		16.7% developed local wound infections
		8.3% with temporal headache
		0% intracranial complications
Gerbino et al,[21] 2000	158	Group 1: Nondisplaced, asymptomatic fractures treated with observation

Group 2: Depressed anterior wall fracture repaired with ORIF

Group 3: Comminuted and dislocated posterior table fractures undergoing cranialization

6.5% meningitis

2.2% frontal bone osteomyelitis

8.7% with frontal deformity

Group 4: NFOT involvement without posterior table fractures treated with stenting of the duct

Abbreviations: CSF, cerebrospinal fluid; NFOT, nasofrontal outflow tract; ORIF, open reduction and internal fixation.

complications leading to eventual death. Regardless of the type of trauma, these patients should be followed over the long term, as it can take up to 25 years for the complications to develop.[19]

SUMMARY

Frontal sinus fractures typically result from high-velocity injuries. Associated injuries are common and can include significant neurologic sequelae. Management options range from observation to an ablative frontal sinus procedure depending on the type of injury. Traditional open approaches remain proven methods for repair, but more recent literature supports the use of endoscopic assistance and minimally invasive preservation techniques for definitive treatment. Regardless of the method chosen for repair, appropriate initial management is important in preventing long-term complications. Given the severity of complications that can develop, these patients should be periodically followed over the long term.

SUPPLEMENTARY DATA

Supplementary data related to this article can be found online at http://doi:10.1016/j.otc.2013.07.005.

REFERENCES

1. Danesh-Sani SA, Bavandi R, Esmaili M. Frontal sinus agenesis using computed tomography. J Craniofac Surg 2011;22(6):e48–51.
2. Rice D. Management of frontal sinus fractures. Curr Opin Otolaryngol Head Neck Surg 2004;12:46–8.
3. Wormald PJ. Endoscopic sinus surgery: anatomy, three-dimensional reconstruction, and surgical technique. New York: Thieme Medical Publishers; 2007. Print.
4. Enepekides D, Donald P. Frontal sinus trauma. In: Stewart M, editor. Head, face, and neck trauma: comprehensive management. New York: Thieme Medical Publishers; 2005. p. 26–39.
5. Nahum A. The biomechanics of maxillofacial trauma. Clin Plast Surg 1975;2(1):59–64.
6. Ioannides C, Freihofer H, Friends J. Fractures of the frontal sinus: a rationale of treatment. Br J Plast Surg 1993;46:208–14.

7. Roden K, Tong W, Surrusco M, et al. Changing characteristics of facial fractures treated at a regional, Level 1 Trauma Center, from 2005-2010: an assessment of patient demographics, referral patterns, etiology of injury, anatomic location, and clinical outcomes. Ann Plast Surg 2012;68(5):461–6.

8. Donald P. The tenacity of the frontal sinus mucosa. Otolaryngol Head Neck Surg 1979;87:557–66.

9. Pollock R, Hill J, Davenport D, et al. Cranialization in a cohort of 154 consecutive patients with frontal sinus fractures (1987-2007): review and update of a compelling procedure in the selected patient. Ann Plast Surg 2013;71(1):54–9.

10. Rodriguez E, Stanwix M, Nam A, et al. Twenty-six-year experience treating frontal sinus fractures: a novel algorithm based on anatomical fracture pattern and failure of conventional techniques. Plast Reconstr Surg 2008;122(6):1850–66.

11. Smith T, Han J, Loehrl T, et al. Endoscopic management of the frontal recess in frontal sinus fractures; a shift in the paradigm? Laryngoscope 2002;112(5):784–90.

12. Lappert P, Lee J. Treatment of an isolated outer table frontal sinus fracture using endoscopic reduction and fixation. Plast Reconstr Surg 1998;102(5):1642–5.

13. Graham H, Spring P. Endoscopic repair of frontal sinus fracture: case report. J Craniomaxillofac Trauma 1996;2:52–5.

14. Kim K, Kim E, Hwang J, et al. Transcutaneous transfrontal approach through a small peri-eyebrow incision for the reduction of closed anterior table frontal sinus fractures. J Plast Reconstr Aesthet Surg 2010;63(5):763–8.

15. Sailer H, Gratz K, Kalavrezos N. Frontal sinus fractures: principles of treatment and long-term results after sinus obliteration with the use of lyophilized cartilage. J Craniomaxillofac Surg 1998;26(4):235–42.

16. Mickel T, Rohrich R, Robinson J. Frontal sinus obliteration: a comparison of fat, muscle, bone, and spontaneous osteoneogenesis in the cat model. Plast Reconstr Surg 1995;95(3):586–92.

17. Rodriquez I, Uceda M, Lobato R, et al. Posttraumatic frontal sinus obliteration with calvarial bone dust and demineralized bone matrix: a long term prospective study and literature review. Int J Oral Maxillofac Surg 2013;42(1):71–6.

18. Rohrich R, Hollier J. Management of frontal sinus fractures. Changing concepts. Clin Plast Surg 1992;19(1):219–32.

19. Wallis A, Donald P. Frontal sinus fractures: a review of 72 cases. Laryngoscope 1988;98:593–8.

20. Oberascher G, Arrer E. Initial clinical experiences with beta 2-transferrin in oto- and rhinorrhea. HNO 1986;34(4):151–5.

21. Gerbino G, Roccia F, Benech A, et al. Analysis of 158 frontal sinus fractures: current surgical management and complications. J Craniomaxillofac Surg 2000;28:133–9.

22. Scholsem M, Scholtes F, Collignon F, et al. Surgical management of anterior cranial base fractures with cerebrospinal fluid fistulae: a single institution experience. Neurosurgery 2008;62:463–71.

23. Brodie H. Prophylactic antibiotics for posttraumatic cerebrospinal fluid fistulae. A meta-analysis. Arch Otolaryngol Head Neck Surg 1997;123(7):749–52.

24. Castro B, Walcott B, Redjal N, et al. Cerebrospinal fluid fistula prevention and treatment following frontal sinus fractures: a review of initial management and outcomes. Neurosurg Focus 2012;32(6):E1.

25. Donald P. Frontal sinus fractures. In: Donald P, editor. The sinuses. New York: Raven Press; 1995. Print.

26. Dhepnorrarat R, Subramaniam S, Sethi D. Endoscopic surgery for fronto-ethmoidal mucoceles: a 15-year experience. Otolaryngol Head Neck Surg 2012;147(2):345–50.

27. Al-Qudah M, Graham S. Modified osteoplastic flap approach for frontal sinus disease. Ann Otol Rhinol Laryngol 2012;121(3):192–6.
28. Chen T, Wang H, Chen S, et al. Reconstruction of post-traumatic frontal-bone depression using hydroxyapatite cement. Ann Plast Surg 2004;52(3):303–8.
29. Choi M, Li Y, Shapiro S, et al. A 10-year review of frontal sinus fractures: clinical outcomes of conservative management of posterior table fractures. Plast Reconstr Surg 2012;130(2):399–406.
30. Tedaldi M, Ramieri V, Foresta E, et al. Experience in the management of frontal sinus fractures. J Craniofac Surg 2010;21(1):208–10.
31. Chen K, Chen C, Mardini S, et al. Frontal sinus fractures: a treatment algorithm and assessment of outcomes based on 78 clinical cases. Plast Reconstr Surg 2006;118(2):457–68.
32. Lakhani R, Shibuya T, Mathog R, et al. Titanium mesh repair of the severely comminuted frontal sinus fracture. Arch Otolaryngol Head Neck Surg 2001;127(6):665–9.

Surgical Treatment of Traumatic Injuries of the Cranial Base

Derrick T. Lin, MD*, Alice C. Lin, MD

KEYWORDS

- Skull base trauma • Craniofacial trauma • Skull base fractures
- Basilar skull fractures • Surgical treatment of skull fractures • CSF leak

KEY POINTS

- Although conservative management may be appropriate for some skull-base injuries, prompt and judicious surgical management can improve morbidity and reduce the risk of meningitis.
- Management of the skull-base fracture depends largely on the type of injury, the location of injury, and the presence or absence of a cerebrospinal fluid (CSF) leak. The presence of a persistent leak is the most common indication for surgical intervention.
- Preoperative studies should include computed tomography with image-guidance navigation and with axial, coronal, and sagittal reconstructions for surgical planning. Other ancillary studies to confirm or locate a CSF leak may be used.
- Preoperative studies to rule out injury to the carotid artery and the need for preoperative endovascular treatment is crucial.
- The anatomy and location of trauma dictates the approach and surgical treatment needed. The high success rate of endoscopic management has greatly reduced the morbidity of skull-base reconstruction and has increased the otolaryngologist's involvement in these interventions.
- Massive tissue loss with multiple comminuted fractures or severe derangements to the skull base may require intracranial repair. Loss of adjacent tissue such as the orbit or skin may require microvascular free-tissue transfer for the best results.

INTRODUCTION

Skull-base fractures (or basilar skull fractures) are potentially devastating fractures of the craniofacial skeleton. These fractures involve 1 or more of the following bones: cribriform plate of the ethmoid bone, orbital plate of the frontal bone, sphenoid bone, occipital bone, or petrous or squamous temporal bone. Although the fracture

Disclosure Statement: Derrick Lin was a one-time consultant for Medtronics (2011). The investigators have no other disclosures or conflicts of interest concerning the contents of this article.
Division of Head and Neck Oncology, Massachusetts Eye and Ear Infirmary, Massachusetts General Hospital, Harvard Medical School, 243 Charles Street, Boston, MA 02114, USA
* Corresponding author.
E-mail address: Derrick_Lin@meei.harvard.edu

themselves only require reduction and reconstruction when the skull base is severely comminuted and altered, even small fractures are associated with shear forces which can create tears in the meninges and thus predispose to cerebrospinal fluid (CSF) leaks. In addition, encephaloceles or meningoencephaloceles can form in these skull-base defects, potentially leading to a surgical emergency.

SIGNS AND SYMPTOMS

Signs and symptoms of skull-base fractures include epistaxis, CSF rhinorrhea, clear otorrhea, periorbital ecchymosis (raccoon eyes), hemotympanum, and ecchymosis of the mastoid process or postauricular area (Battle sign). Other signs are manifestations of cranial nerve or sensory deficits such as ophthalmoplegia, deafness, nystagmus, or other cranial nerve palsies. The first, third, fifth and seventh cranial nerves are the most common to present with palsies.[1,2]

CSF Leak

The diagnosis of a CSF leak may be obvious, such as the patient with profuse clear drainage that is reproducible with positioning. However, more often the diagnosis is confounded by the similar appearance of nasal secretions and a more intermittent leak.

Described signs of CSF leak include the reservoir sign or flexing of the head to elicit CSF, and the target sign or a bull's-eye stain, with blood in the center when drainage is collected on gauze or a napkin. This sign is caused by a further migration of CSF than blood, but is unreliable because nasal secretions can create the same pattern. Both of these signs have unknown, but not particularly high sensitivities or specificities.[3]

CSF leak with possible resultant meningitis is the major complication of skull-base trauma, and results from even minor tears in the dura during impact. Head injuries associated with craniofacial fractures are the cause of 80% of CSF leaks, and CSF leaks develop in 11% to 45% of skull fractures.[2,3] CSF leaks resulting from trauma usually begin within 48 hours of injury and are apparent within 3 months 95% of the time. More than 70% of these leaks cease with conservative nonsurgical treatment, which includes bed rest and CSF diversion.[4] The mechanism of the resolution of the leak is unknown but is thought to be due to regeneration of the nasal mucosa or fibrous tissue. The location of the trauma may dictate whether a CSF leak is likely to close spontaneously with conservative measures. For example, the geometry of the skull base at the cribriform plate is unfavorable for spontaneous resolution of a leak. In other areas, mild herniation of the brain can create a seal to close the leak, but this is difficult to achieve at the cribriform plate.

ASSESSMENT
Laboratory Studies

The β2-transferrin test is the most popular chemical test for CSF leaks, as β2-transferrin is a protein that is found only in CSF, perilymph, and aqueous humor. The presence of β2-transferrin in nasal secretions is accurate for diagnosing CSF leaks, with 99% sensitivity and 97% specificity. However, there are often errors in interpretation and there is a lag time in the results, as the assays take 1 to 2 days to perform. Although only 0.5 mL is needed, this can be difficult to obtain in small intermittent leaks. Alternatives to β2-transferrin testing are using comparison testing of glucose, electrolytes, and protein with the serum and the use of β-trace protein (BTP). Testing of glucose, electrolytes, and protein is easy and rapid, but there can be many confounding factors. BTP is not readily available at many institutions but constitutes a faster test than β2-transferrin. BTP is not as accurate as β2-transferrin because it is not as specific for CSF.[4,5]

Intrathecal Injection

Intrathecal fluorescein can be used for an accuracy of 96% when wide skull-base exposure has already been obtained or will be obtained.[4] However, although rare, the complications of fluorescein can range from tinnitus, headaches, nausea, and vomiting to pulmonary edema, confusion, seizures, coma, and even death. Therefore, its use requires a thorough informed consent with explanation of the risks to the patient. Intrathecal fluorescein has not been approved by the Food and Drug Administration. Complications from intrathecal fluorescein mainly result from an error in the administration, as many studies have shown reliable safety in the small dose that is adequate for a preoperative examination. Schlosser and Bolger[4] found no complications when using 0.1 mL of 10% fluorescein diluted in 10 mL of the patient's CSF and a slow injection over 10 to 15 minutes. Similarly, other investigators have reported other formulations and dilutions of fluorescein that have produced no complications.

Imaging

High-resolution computed tomography (HRCT) with axial, coronal, and sagittal reconstruction is an important study in preoperative planning for the definition of bony details needed to plan the optimal approach.[6–8] It also has 87% accuracy in predicting traumatic CSF leaks,[7] but cannot always define its exact location. Coronal cuts may be able to provide the most information regarding the location (**Fig. 1**).[2]

Carotid angiography is an important preoperative examination in skull-base trauma, because of the possibility of carotid pseudoaneurysms and carotid-cavernous fistulas. These entities should be ruled out before a surgical approach is attempted.

Pseudoaneurysms and fistulas may be treated in an endovascular fashion before surgical intervention. Computed tomography (CT) cisternography can be useful in identifying the location of a leak in a specific circumstance, although it is more invasive than conventional imaging. Cisternography is currently rarely used, owing to the high quality of information obtained from HRCT.[6,8] Cisternography requires an active leak at the time of intrathecal contrast injection or a reproducible leak by Valsalva, and is most accurate in the frontal and sphenoid sinuses because these sinuses can collect

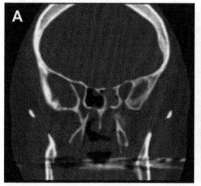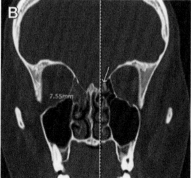

Fig. 1. (*A*) Coronal reconstruction on high-resolution computed tomography (HRCT) of a patient with a basilar skull fracture in the area of the sphenoid. The bony defect and filling of the sinus with fluid is seen. (*B*) Coronal reconstruction on HRCT of a patient with bilateral basilar skull fractures with bony displacement (*arrow*).

and retain the contrast material for a longer period of time to allow capture in the imaging.[4] Radioisotopes can be used in low-flow leaks with the placement of intranasal pledgets typically at the cribriform plate, the middle meatus, and sphenoethmoidal recess, as the pledgets can be left in place for hours. However, this method cannot determine the location of the leak, and can have low sensitivity and high false-positive rates.[4,7]

Magnetic resonance imaging (MRI) is a technique that uses the hyperintensity of CSF on T2-weighted imaging, and provides helpful additional information regarding the anatomy of the fracture. MRI with fast spin-echo sequence, fat suppression, and image reversal can have accuracy up to 89%. MRI can be similar to CT cisternography, but has the advantage of being noninvasive and also has the ability to differentiate brain parenchyma from CSF[5]; however, high false-positive rates have also been reported.

NONSURGICAL MANAGEMENT OF SKULL-BASE FRACTURES

Although the focus of this review is the surgical management of skull-base fractures, determining the need for surgery is a salient and well-debated topic. Investigators agree that a good proportion of fractures do not need surgical treatment, and many CSF leaks resolve with conservative management. Fifty percent to 85% of posttraumatic CSF leaks close spontaneously within 1 week.[2,6,9,10] Nonsurgical management entails bed rest with head-of-bed elevation, carbonic anhydrase inhibitors, and strict precautions against CSF leak such as prevention of straining, nose blowing, use of straws, Valsalva maneuvers, and incentive spirometers.[11,12] If noninterventional techniques fail, CSF diversion with lumbar drain puncture or a ventriculostomy tube is another useful tool.[3,6] Although a large portion of posttraumatic CSF leaks resolve with nonoperative management, this does not indicate that the dura has sealed,[13,14] and these patients should be counseled and followed for recurrent CSF leaks or late meningoencephaloceles.[15-17] Delayed CSF leaks require operative management, as the chance of spontaneous cessation is low[17,18] and these patients have a high risk of meningitis.[14,18,19]

SURGICAL MANAGEMENT OF SKULL-BASE FRACTURES

Surgical treatment is indicated for fractures associated with CSF leaks that do not close with conservative management, or trauma with significant tissue loss and anatomic distortion. The general approach to repair is identifying the region that requires repair, preparation of the recipient area, and accurate placement of graft material. Surgical management has been shown to reduce the incidence of meningitis from 30% to 4% in the acute setting. The long-term benefits are even more marked, with a reduction from 85% to 7% 10 years after injury.[13,14]

Timing of Surgery

For small to moderate posttraumatic CSF leaks, it may be reasonable to wait 72 hours to 1 week before surgical intervention, thus allowing time for stabilization of the patient and also allowing the opportunity for spontaneous sealing of the leak. However, the clinician should be mindful of the risk of meningitis, which is 0.62% within the first day of injury and increases by 7% to 9% per week for the first 2 weeks.[14] The architecture of the fracture and the skull base can dictate the necessity for early repair. Significant trauma with multiple comminuted fractures, large fractures, severely depressed fractures, encephalocele, or large CSF leaks would dictate earlier repair because they are unlikely to heal.[20-23] Leaks near the midline or in the cribriform plate also are more likely to require surgical repair. In the setting of need for emergent surgery for other intracranial abnormality such as tension pneumocephalus or evacuation of hematoma, a dural repair can be performed at the same time as the craniotomy, as long as the neurologic status is good and there is no concern for intracranial edema.[1,2,20,21]

Some investigators advocate surgical repair without a trial of conservative management for more than 1 cm of bony displacement, midline fractures, and involvement of the cribriform plate, because of the smaller chance of spontaneous healing in these cases.[11,14] It is the authors' opinion that the decision for conservative management rather than surgical repair is dictated by multiple patient factors and cannot follow hard and fast rules.

Transcranial Approach

Dandy[20] first described the transcranial approach in 1926. Success rates of open repair have been shown to be approximately 70% in the past,[23,24] but one series published great results with the use of vascularized fascia and fibrin glue and a success rate of 100%.[9] This approach creates wide exposure of the fracture area but is associated with significant morbidity and complications. Nevertheless, when fractures require neurosurgical intervention for other intracranial processes, this approach is a good option as the dural repair can be performed concurrently.

Extracranial Approach

The major recent improvement in the extracranial approach is the use of endoscopic sinus surgery to repair CSF leaks. Endoscopic repair has become a new favored method of repair because of its lower morbidity and high success rates. Endoscopic repair is especially useful for small defects in the sphenoid, cribriform, and ethmoid roof.[25,26] Success rates of 94% to 100% have been reported.[23–28] The endoscopic approach depends largely on the likely location of the leak. General considerations include a wide exposure of the injury, tailoring the approach to the location of injury, and use of judicious antiseptic techniques. Mucosa surrounding the bony defect should be removed to expose the edges of the defect and create a bare bony rim for the onlay graft to seal to the bone, thus closing off the defect. Inlay grafts of bone or cartilage can also be used. Encephaloceles can be ablated using bipolar cautery. Endoscopic bipolar cautery devices can be used to reach less accessible sites, thus avoiding monopolar cautery with its risks to the optic nerve and orbital contents. Meticulous hemostasis must be obtained to avoid intracranial hemorrhage, especially at the base of the encephalocele. Once the defect is closed off from the extracranial cavity, any bleeding becomes an intracranial collection and thus a risk for intracranial injury.[4,29]

Lateral Skull-Base Fractures

Temporal bone fractures with skull-base involvement rarely require surgical intervention. The most common need for intervention is for injury to the facial nerve, described in Boahene's chapter on the management of the facial nerve after trauma elsewhere in this issue. Other emergent indications for surgical repair include encephaloceles into the middle ear, mastoid, or external auditory meatus, or for control of hemorrhage. Surgery for control of hemorrhage should be performed in conjunction with endovascular techniques. In the setting of an encephalocele into the mastoid or middle ear, the surgical approach starts with a wide mastoidectomy. Once the meningocele is localized, the surrounding bone should be removed with a diamond burr. Meningoceles and herniated brain can be treated with bipolar electrocautery, as herniated brain is likely dysfunctional.[15,16,30,31] Dural repair can be performed with suturing or graft material, and abdominal fat is commonly used for bolstering the repair and filling the defect. Semaan and colleagues[30] advocate the use of a cartilage graft placed in an epidural pocket created by elevation of the dura surrounding the bony defect. In their series of 31 consecutive patients they reported a failure rate of 0%.

Ethmoid roof and cribriform fractures

This area is readily accessible via an endoscopic approach. The surgical approach requires a careful and complete anterior ethmoidectomy, and middle and superior turbinectomies to expose the fracture and area of leak.[29] Once the area requiring repair is determined, adjacent sinuses should be opened to prevent the development of a postoperative mucocele and to increase the exposure for the repair. The dura can be elevated off above the bony-skull defect to create a potential space for the inlay graft. Bone is optimal for inlay grafts, as it creates rigid support to prevent recurrent encephalocele.

Grafts can be taken from bone fragments found during the approach, middle turbinate bone, or from thinned calvarial bone grafts that may be available from adjunctive procedures, and meticulously fashioned into the correct size and shape. Fascial grafts or free mucosal grafts used in an onlay fashion are appropriate for a second layer of closure.[4,6]

Sphenoid fractures

Endoscopic transethmoid approaches with a wide sphenoidotomy can be used as the initial approach. In this case, removal of adjacent mucosa may not be as wide as more anterior locations, owing to the proximity of the carotid and optic nerves. Obliteration of the entire sphenoid sinus is not recommended because of the risk to these structures when attempting a full evacuation of sphenoid mucosa for the obliteration. Graft materials for repair include fascia, bone, and synthetic materials. Autologous fat is another good option for a primary graft material for a small defect or as a secondary onlay to bolster and support the graft. Abdominal fat can act as biological packing and, once involution occurs, will not cause obliteration of the sinus or mucocele formation.

After this initial approach, fractures found to be involving the lateral recess of the sphenoid may require a transpterygoid approach. A wide maxillary antrostomy is performed and the posterior wall of the maxillary sinus is removed. The internal maxillary artery and its branches should be identified and either ligated or moved out of the field. Care should be taken to preserve cranial nerves V2, the vidian nerve, and the sphenopalatine ganglion; this allows access to the lateral-anterior wall of the sphenoid sinus, which should be reduced using a drill to create the exposure needed to repair lateral sphenoid defects.[4]

Frontal sinus fractures

Surgical management of frontal sinus fractures is described in detail in the article by Brissett elsewhere in this issue.

Choosing graft materials and packing

Graft materials include bone, cartilage, pericranium, fascia lata, temporalis muscle fascia, or other autologous or nonautologous grafts. Bone can be harvested from the fracture or from mastoid, septum, turbinate, or cadaveric bone.[4,29] The size of the defect and the amount of strain on the repair dictates the need for more firm graft material or multilayered repair. Hegazy and colleagues found inlay and onlay grafting to have similar results. The overlay technique requires adhesive such as fibrin glue, which has been shown to increase graft adherence and the strength of the repair.

The purpose of packing is to separate the repair from the rest of the sinonasal tract and the negative pressures that can be created. Using multiple layers of nonadherent packing, such as Silastic or Gelfilm, may prevent shear forces or frictional movement and disruption of the graft. Packing should be removed after 1 week when the graft has adhered to the repair site.

MASSIVE TRAUMATIC INJURIES TO THE SKULL BASE

Massive traumatic injuries to the skull base with multiple, comminuted defects and badly attenuated skull bases may require an intracranial approach, consisting of neurosurgical intervention with craniotomy and dural repair, with an additional layer of vascularized coverage such as a pericranial flap or a temporalis fascial graft.[1] In cases of massive traumatic injury with loss of adjacent tissue, free-flap reconstruction has become the most favorable method of reconstruction because it can be used to create a vascularized repair of the skull base as well as fill in the defect of adjacent tissue loss. The most common adjacent tissue loss requiring free-flap reconstruction is the loss of skin or the need to remove a dysfunctional orbit. Radial forearm, anterolateral thigh, rectus, and latissimus free flaps can be good options depending on the volume and area of adjacent tissue loss. Free-flap reconstruction can also be considered in cases of multiple failed repairs and lack of adjacent vascularized tissue.

Lumbar Drain

The use of a lumbar drain in the postoperative setting relies on the anecdotal concept of decreasing the CSF pressure and stress on the repair. However, many studies have not found a difference in rates of repair failure with use of a lumbar drain, which may be due to the high underlying success rates of skull-base repair. In the authors' opinion, insertion of a lumbar drain for posttraumatic repair is not necessary.

Antibiotics

The use of antibiotics in the setting of posttraumatic CSF leaks has been a controversial topic. Its use is encouraged by the significant risk of meningitis; however, multiple retrospective studies have shown no difference in the incidence of meningitis with the use of antibiotics.[1,21,32–34] Future prospective controlled and randomized trials may be needed to further investigate the topic, but for the meantime arguments against antibiotics include no known difference in meningitis rates as well as, possibly, colonization with resistant strains of bacteria and inability to eradicate bacterial colonization of the "dirty" sinonasal cavity. Studies have discovered an increase in the rate of meningitis in the immediate period after antibiotics are stopped.[33,34]

COMPLICATIONS OF SKULL-BASE SURGERY

Complications include:

- Meningitis
- Recurrent leak or failure of repair
- Sinusitis
- Visual disturbances
- Seizures
- Pneumocephalus
- Intracranial hypertension
- Cavernous sinus thrombosis

The risk of meningitis after a traumatic CSF leak is 5% to 50%, and there is a neurologic complication rate of approximately 30%.[1,13,14] There is a 1.3% risk per day in the first 2 weeks after injury, 7.4% in the first month, and 85% within 10 years. Operative mortality is 1.3% to 24.9%, and recurrence of CSF leak occurs in 2% to 20%.[14] Recurrences after a second repair are rare.[1] Pneumocephalus is another devastating complication that requires vigilant attention. In patients with lumbar drains, the drain must be kept open in the immediate postoperative period, even during extubation or movement, to ensure that Valsalva or increases in pressure during this time do not lead to life-threatening pneumocephalus. There is an albeit small but real risk of major complications such as seizures, cavernous sinus thrombosis, intracranial hypertension, and death.

REFERENCES

1. Scholsem M, Scholtes F, Collignon F, et al. Surgical management of anterior cranial base fractures with cerebrospinal fluid fistulae: a single-institution experience. Neurosurgery 2008;2:463–71.
2. Yilmazlar S, Arslan E, Kocaeli H, et al. Cerebrospinal fluid leakage complicating skull base fractures: analysis of 81 cases. Neurosurg Rev 2006;29:64–71.
3. Ziu M, Savage JG, Jimenez DF. Diagnosis and treatment of cerebrospinal fluid rhinorrhea following accidental traumatic skull base fractures. Neurosurg Focus 2012;32(6):E3.
4. Schlosser RJ, Bolger WE. Nasal cerebrospinal fluid leaks: critical review and surgical considerations. Laryngoscope 2004;114:255–65.
5. Eljamel MS. The role of surgery and B2-transferrin in the management of CSF fistulas [MD thesis]. Liverpool (United Kingdom): University of Liverpool; 1993. p. 207–19.
6. Bell RB, Dierks EJ, Homer L, et al. Management of cerebrospinal fluid leak associated with craniomaxillofacial trauma. J Oral Maxillofac Surg 2004;62: 676–84.
7. Zapalac JS, Marple BF, Schwade ND. Skull base cerebrospinal fluid fistulas: a comprehensive diagnostic algorithm. Otolaryngol Head Neck Surg 2002;126: 669–76.
8. Eljamel MS, Pidgeon CN. Localization of inactive cerebrospinal fluid fistula. J Neurosurg 1995;83:795–8.
9. Mincy JE. Posttraumatic cerebrospinal fluid fistula of the frontal fossa. J Trauma 1966;6:618–22.
10. Passagia JG, Chirossel JP, Favre JJ, et al. Surgical approaches to the anterior fossa and preservation of olfaction. In: Cohadon F, editor. Advances and technical standard in neurosurgery, vol. 25. Wein (Austria): Springer; 1999. p. 197–241.
11. Rocchi G, Caroli E, Belli E, et al. Severe craniofacial fractures with frontobasal involvement and cerebrospinal fluid fistula: indications for surgical repair. Surg Neurol 2005;63:559–64.
12. Zuckreman JD, DelGaudio JM. Utility of preoperative high-resolution CT and intraoperative image guidance in identification of cerebrospinal fluid leaks for endoscopic repair. Am J Rhinol 2008;22:151–4.
13. Eljamel MS, Foy PM. Acute traumatic CSF fistulae: the risk of intracranial infection. Br J Neurosurg 1990;4:381–5.
14. Eljamel MS, Foy PM. Post-traumatic CSF fistulae, the case for surgical repair. Br J Neurosurg 1990;4:479–82.

15. Jackson CG, Pappas DG Jr, Manolidis S, et al. Brain herniation into the middle ear and mastoid: concepts in diagnosis and surgical management. Am J Otol 1997;18:198–205.
16. Kamerer DB, Caparosa J. Temporal bone encephalocele—diagnosis and treatment. Laryngoscope 1982;92(8 Pt 1):878–82.
17. Manelfe C, Cellerier P, Sobel D, et al. Cerebrospinal fluid rhinorrhea: evaluation with metrizamide cisternography. AJR Am J Roentgenol 1982;138:471–6.
18. Talamonti G, Fontana RA, Villa F, et al. "High risk" anterior basal skull fractures. Surgical treatment of 64 consecutive cases. J Neurosurg Sci 1995;39:191–7.
19. Park JI, Strelzow VV, Friedman WH. Current management of cerebrospinal fluid rhinorrhea. Laryngoscope 1983;93:1294–300.
20. Dandy WE. Pneumocephalus (intracranial pneumatocele or aerocoele). Arch Surg 1926;12:949–82.
21. Comoy J. Craniofacial injuries. Neurosurgical problems. J Neuroradiol 1986;13: 248–52.
22. Sakas DE, Beale DJ, Ameen AA, et al. Compound anterior cranial base fractures: classification using computerized tomography scanning as a basis for selection of patients for dural repair. J Neurosurg 1998;88:471–7.
23. Lanza DC, O'Brien DA, Kennedy DW. Endoscopic repair of cerebrospinal fluid fistulae and encephaloceles. Laryngoscope 1996;106:1119–25.
24. Schick B, Ibing R, Brors D, et al. Long-term study of endonasal duraplasty and review of the literatures. Ann Otol Rhinol Laryngol 2001;110:142–7.
25. Kirtane MV, Gautham K, Upadhyaya SR. Endoscopic CSF rhinorrhea closure: our experience in 267 cases. Otolaryngol Head Neck Surg 2005;132:208–12.
26. McMains KC, Gross CW, Kountakis SE. Endoscopic management of cerebrospinal fluid rhinorrhea. Laryngoscope 2004;114:1833–7.
27. Banks CA, Palmer JN, Chiu AG, et al. Endoscopic closure of CSF rhinorrhea: 193 cases over 21 years. Otolaryngol Head Neck Surg 2009;130:826–33.
28. Cassano M, Felippu A. Endoscopic treatment of cerebrospinal fluid leaks with the use of lower turbinate grafts: a retrospective review of 125 cases. Rhinology 2009;47:362–8.
29. Kim E, Russel PT. Prevention and management of skull base injury. Otolaryngol Clin North Am 2010;43:809–16.
30. Semaan MT, Gilpin DA, Hsu DP, et al. Transmastoid extradural-intracranial approach for repair of transtemporal meningoencephalocele: a review of 31 consecutive cases. Laryngoscope 2011;121:1765–72.
31. Patel A, Groppo E. Management of temporal bone trauma. Craniomaxillofac Trauma Reconstr 2010;3:105–13.
32. Eljamel MS. Antibiotic prophylaxis in the management of CSF fistula. Surg Neurol 1998;50:387.
33. Greig JR. Antibiotic prophylaxis after CSF leaks lacks evidence base. BMJ 2002; 32:1037.
34. Ratilal B, Costa J, Sampaio C. Antibiotic prophylaxis for preventing meningitis in patients with basilar skull fractures. Cochrane Database Syst Rev 2006;(1):CD004884.

Surgical Management of Complex Midfacial Fractures

Amit Kochhar, MD[a], Patrick J. Byrne, MD[b],*

KEYWORDS

- Trauma • Midface fracture • Orbit • Zygomaticomaxillary complex
- Naso-orbital-ethmoid • Le Fort fracture

KEY POINTS

- The midface is composed of several paired vertical buttresses and horizontal buttresses that protect vital organs, such as the brain, optic nerves, and brainstem. Damage to the midfacial buttress system causes functional and cosmetic deformity.
- High impact trauma to the midface causes complex fracture patterns. These include zygomaticomaxilary complex, orbital wall and floor, naso-orbital-ethmoid, and Le Fort fractures.
- Diagnosis of midfacial fractures requires a thorough physical examination and high-resolution computed tomography scanning.
- The goal of surgical treatment is to restore the bony infrastructure of the midface while disrupting the least amount of soft tissue.

INTRODUCTION

The craniofacial skeleton is designed to support and protect critical organs, such as the eyes, optic nerves, brain, and brainstem. This is especially true of the midface, which consists of the paired zygomas, orbits, maxilla, and nasal bones. Each of these components is susceptible to complex fractures with high-impact injury. Distinct patterns, such as the zygomaticomaxillary complex (ZMC), orbital, naso-orbital-ethmoid (NOE) complex, and Le Fort–type fracture, occur with blunt trauma and result in cosmetic and functional deformity. Diagnosis requires a thorough physical examination and high-resolution computed tomography (CT) scanning. Depending on the

Disclosures: The authors have no disclosures.
Conflict of Interest: The authors have no conflicts of interest.
[a] Department of Otolaryngology, Head and Neck Surgery, Johns Hopkins School of Medicine, 601 North, Caroline Street 6th Floor, Baltimore, MD 21287, USA; [b] Division of Facial Plastic and Reconstructive Surgery, Johns Hopkins School of Medicine, 601 North, Caroline Street 6th Floor, Baltimore, MD 21287, USA
* Corresponding author.
E-mail address: pbyrne2@jhmi.edu

Otolaryngol Clin N Am 46 (2013) 759–778
http://dx.doi.org/10.1016/j.otc.2013.06.002
0030-6665/13/$ – see front matter Published by Elsevier Inc.

oto.theclinics.com

amount of displacement or bone loss, treatment may vary from simple observation to open reduction and fixation. The goal of treatment is to restore the bony infrastructure to achieve optimal reduction while disrupting the least amount of soft tissue.

The midface can be described as several paired vertical (nasomaxillary or medial, zygomaticomaxillary or lateral, and pterygomaxillary or posterior) and horizontal buttresses (frontal bone and supraorbital rims, nasal bones and inferior orbital rims, and the hard palate) (**Fig. 1**). The thicker vertical buttresses resist functional stresses (biting), whereas the thinner horizontal buttresses protect organs and define facial shape, but are relatively weak and collapse on impact.[1–3] Restoration of the facial buttresses is an important concept in fracture management. Priority is given to disrupted buttresses to restore facial height (vertical buttresses) and projection (horizontal buttresses). Complex fractures of the midface may result in cosmetic and functional deformity. Thus, there are two aspects to consider during repair. First, there must be proper realignment of the bones to recreate aesthetic form and occlusal function. Second, a systematic fixation must be accomplished through rigid fixation by plates and screws. This fixation is designed to maximize the amount of stability created at the time of repair to minimize callus formation, infection, and any shifting in the surgical positioning.[4,5] The challenge for the reconstructive surgeon is to restore patients to their preinjury form and function. New developments and improved understanding of fracture management have significantly improved outcomes. This article explores surgical approaches and techniques for repair of complex midfacial fractures.

OVERVIEW

The body of the zygoma forms the malar prominence. It is an important aesthetic feature and is also the most anterior projection of the lateral face, thus at high risk

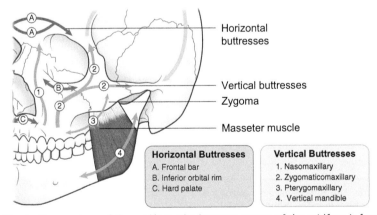

Horizontal Buttresses	Vertical Buttresses
A. Frontal bar	1. Nasomaxillary
B. Inferior orbital rim	2. Zygomaticomaxillary
C. Hard palate	3. Pterygomaxillary
	4. Vertical mandible

Fig. 1. The buttress system of the midface. The buttress system of the midface is formed by the frontal, maxillary, zygomatic, and sphenoid bones and their articulations to one another. The vertical buttresses are composed by the medial nasomaxillary buttress, the lateral zygomaticomaxillary buttress, and the posterior pterygomaxillary buttress. Three horizontal buttresses interconnect and provide support for the vertical buttresses. These are the (1) frontal bone and supraorbital rims, (2) the nasal bones and inferior orbital rims, and (3) the hard palate. (*Adapted from* Linnau KF, Stanley RB Jr., Hallam DK, et al. Imaging of high-energy midfacial trauma: what the surgeon needs to know. Eur J Radiol 2003;48:17–32; with permission.)

for injury. The strong zygoma serves two purposes. First, it is the attachment for the powerful masseter muscle, which is essential to mastication. Second, the zygoma serves as the cornerstone of support for the vertical buttress system of the midface (see **Fig. 1**). The bones that articulate with the zygoma tend to be weaker and trauma often results in fractures at its suture lines: the zygomaticofrontal superiorly, the zygomaticotemporal posterolaterally, the zygomaticomaxillary medially, and the zygomaticosphenoid posteriorly (**Fig. 2**).[6] These fractures are called ZMC fractures, and often tripod fractures; however, if all four sutures are involved, these fractures should be referred to as tetrapod fractures.

ZMC fractures are the second most common type of facial fracture in patients with blunt trauma after only nasal bone fractures. Because the amount of force applied to the fracture site differs, the amount of displacement and bone loss also vary. Thus, a broad spectrum of fracture patterns range from isolated nondisplaced zygoma fractures to severely displaced and comminuted ZMC components.[7] There are several classification systems used to describe ZMC fractures. The Zingg classification (**Table 1**) system groups them into three categories (A, B, and C).[8] Type A injuries, the least common, are isolated to one component of the tetrapod fracture. They are further subclassified into A1 for zygomatic arch fractures, A2 for lateral orbital wall fractures, and A3 for inferior orbital wall fractures. Types B and C account for more than 60% of ZMC injuries.[9] Type B fractures involve injury to all four of the supporting structures, and type C fractures are complex fractures with comminution of the zygomatic bone.

The zygoma is intricately associated with the orbit and with the exception of isolated zygomatic arch fractures, always include a component of the orbital floor (**Fig. 3**).[6] Inferomedially, the zygoma extends from the inferior orbital rim and broadly contacts the maxilla by the zygomaticomaxillary suture line to form another vertical buttress (see **Fig. 1**). The zygoma also contributes to the lateral and inferior orbital rims and the inferolateral orbital walls.[10] Thus, minor displacement of the zygoma can

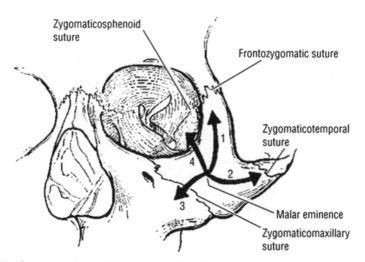

Fig. 2. The four suture lines of the zygomaxillary (ZMC) complex. The bones that articulate with the zygoma tend to be weaker and trauma often results in fractures at its suture lines: (1) the zygomaticofrontal superiorly, (2) the zygomaticotemporal posterolaterally, (3) the zygomaticomaxillary medially, and (4) the zygomaticosphenoid posteriorly. (*From* Strong B, Sykes J. Zygoma complex fracture. Facial Plast Surg 1998;14(1):105–15; with permission.)

Table 1		
Classification systems for complex midface fractures		
Zingg classification for ZMC fractures		
A		
A1	Isolated zygomatic arch fractures	
A2	Isolated lateral orbital wall fractures	
A3	Isolated inferior orbital wall fractures	
B	Injury to all four suture lines	
C	Comminution of the zygomatic bone	
Markowitz and Manson classification for NOE fractures		
Type 1	Single noncomminuted central fragment without medial canthal tendon disruption.	
Type 2	Comminution of the central fragment, but the medial canthal tendon remains firmly attached to a definable segment of bone.	
Type 3	Severe central fragment comminution with disruption of the medial canthal tendon insertion.	
Le Fort fracture classification (all three involve the pterygoid bone)		
I	Transverse maxillary fracture. Fracture line separates the teeth from the upper face. Fracture line passes through the alveolar ridge, lateral nose, and inferior wall of maxillary sinus.	
II	Pyramidal fracture, with the teeth at the pyramid base, and nasofrontal suture at its apex. The fracture arch passes through posterior alveolar ridge, lateral walls of maxillary sinuses, inferior orbital rim, and nasal bones.	
III	Craniofacial disjunction. The fracture line passes through nasofrontal suture, maxillofrontal suture, orbital wall, and zygomatic arch.	

significantly alter the position of the globe in the orbit and significantly impact the anteroposterior position of the globe. External impact to this area may cause orbital wall or floor defects.[11,12] If the orbital rim remains intact, but the force of impact is transmitted to the bones of the floor, roof, and medial wall, an orbital "blowout" fracture results. In

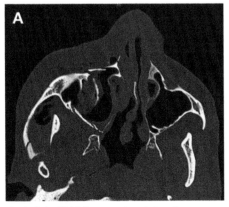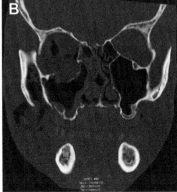

Fig. 3. A right ZMC fracture involving the zygoma, maxilla, orbital floor, and lateral orbital wall. (*A*) Axial CT scan depicting the zygoma, anterior maxilla, and lateral orbital wall fractures with herniation of contents into the maxillary sinus. (*B*) Coronal CT scan depicting the lateral orbital wall, orbital floor, and maxilla fractures with enlargement of the orbital volume relative to the left side.

this case, the continuity of the inferior, lateral, and superior orbital rims remains intact; however, the force is transmitted to the weakest bones, usually the floor and medial wall (**Fig. 4**). Diplopia is the most frequent complication of orbital floor defects. Others include limitation of ocular movement, infraorbital numbness, enophthalmos, and reduced vision or blindness.

The medial orbital wall is composed of the frontal process of the maxilla, the lacrimal bone, the orbital plate of the ethmoid bone, and the sphenoid body. The thin lamina papyracea separates the orbit from the ethmoidal sinuses and is easily damaged. The lacrimal sac lies anteriorly in the lacrimal groove formed by the maxilla and lacrimal bone. At the junction of the medial wall and orbital roof are the anterior and posterior ethmoidal foramina. The anterior and posterior ethmoidal arteries and nerves travel here and may contribute to intraoperative bleeding if not protected during repair. The medial rectus muscle is also closely associated with the medial orbital wall. An obvious sign of medial wall fracture is injury or entrapment to the medial rectus, which presents as reduced adduction or abduction. The medial canthal tendon, trochlea, and lacrimal drainage system are other important structures located medially in the orbit and are susceptible to injury with medial wall trauma.

The orbital floor comprises the maxillary, zygomatic, and palatine bones. The floor terminates at the posterior edge of the maxillary sinus. The inferior rectus muscle, which lies adjacent to the orbital floor, may become involved in fractures of the floor with subsequent motility disturbance. Beneath the floor in the maxilla is the infraorbital foramen, which transmits the maxillary branch of the trigeminal nerve (V2); thus, sensory deficit for the middle of the face often accompanies injury to the orbital floor.

It is important to understand the complex shape of the globe because its contents influence its position. Inferolaterally, the orbital floor is concave; however, medially it is more convex and becomes significantly convex posteriorly at the apex.[5] The greater wing of the sphenoid forms the orbit posterolaterally and the lesser wing contributes to the optic canal posteromedially. Although the location of the optic canal protects it from most injuries, the optic foramen does travel toward the lateral orbital rim. Thus,

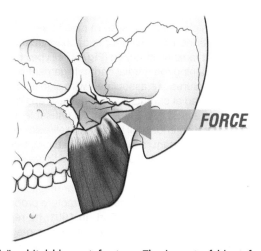

Fig. 4. The "classic" orbital blowout fracture. The impact of blunt force, compresses the contents of the orbit so the path of least resistance for the periorbital tissue is by fracture of the floor and herniation into the maxillary sinus. (*Adapted from* Stack BC, Ruggiero FP. Maxillary and periorbital fractures. In: Baily BJ, Johnson JT, Newlands SD, editors. Head and neck surgery – otolaryngology. 4th edition. Philadelphia: Lippincott Williams & Wilkins; 2006. p. 975–93.)

laterally directed forces may contribute to blindness or visual impairment. The apex of the orbit includes the area lateral to the optic canal and houses cranial nerves III, IV, V, and VI as they enter the orbit. Compression of this area, the superior orbital fissure, causes dysfunction in these nerves, and is an ophthalmologic emergency.[13,14]

The nasal bones are prominently positioned in the middle of the face. Deep to the nasal bones lie the ethmoid sinuses and the medial orbital walls. High-force trauma is transmitted through the nasal bones adjacent to the laminae papyracea and orbit. These provide little support and "crumple" on impact, thus allowing the nasal bones to telescope posteriorly while scattering the compressive wave into the ethmoid sinuses. The ability of these bones to crumple under high impact protects deeper vital structures, such as the brain and optic nerve, and illustrates the advantageous biomechanical design of this region.[15,16]

NOE fractures are the most complex fractures of the face diagnostically and therapeutically. Delayed or inadequate treatment of this region results in deformity that can be only partially corrected, such as a shortened and retruded nose, shortened palpebral fissures, telecanthus, enopthalmos, epiphora, and ocular dystopia.[17–20] The concept of the "central face" refers to injury in which the trauma to the solid nasal root is transmitted posteriorly resulting in a telescoping injury and nasal retrusion.[21] The "central face" includes the attachments for the medial eyelids and the projection of the nose. The medial eyelids are attached by the medial canthal ligaments to the bone of the anterior and posterior lacrimal crests. When these are disrupted, the tendons are pulled laterally (and anteriorly and inferiorly), and the horizontal length of the eyelids is shortened leading to telecanthus (increased distance between the medial canthi, with normal interpupillary distance). Orbital hypertelorism, by contrast, is a congenital increase in the distance between the globes. This needs to be reconstructed adequately to withstand the constant lateral tension of the lids. Epiphora results from obstruction or disruption of any member of the lacrimal outflow system, which is closely related to the medial canthal tendon and the lacrimal and maxillary bones.[15,21–23] Treatment is difficult, because persistent posttraumatic epiphora has been reported in almost one-third of patient's with NOE fractures.[23]

Numerous classification schemes have been used to describe NOE fractures. Markowitz and Manson created a classification system (see **Table 1**) that is based on the status of the medial canthal tendon and the degree of comminution of the fragment of lacrimal crest bone to which it remains attached (**Fig. 5**).[24] Type I fractures occur when a large central fragment containing the medial canthal ligament is separated from the surrounding bone. Type II fractures are associated with significant comminution, but the fragment containing the medial canthal ligament is still repairable. In type III fractures, the tendon is either detached or attached to an unusable fragment.

The maxilla extends from the anterior skull base to the alveolar ridge. Each maxilla is functionally and cosmetically important to the midface because together they form the medial portions of the infraorbital rims and anterior orbital floors and also provide support for the nasal bones. They also form the piriform apertures, and house the maxillary sinuses, nasolacrimal ducts, and dentition important for mastication.

Much of the understanding of patterns of maxillary fracture propagation in midfacial trauma originates from the work of René Le Fort. In 1901, he reported his work on cadaver skulls that were subjected to blunt forces of various magnitudes and directions. He concluded that there are predictable patterns of fractures after blunt injury (see **Table 1**). These fractures occur along three lines of weakness inherent in the design of the facial skeleton (**Fig. 6**).[25] Le Fort I fractures are known as the horizontal maxillary fracture and occur above the level of the maxillary dentition, separating the alveoli and teeth from the remaining craniofacial skeleton. Type I fractures cross the

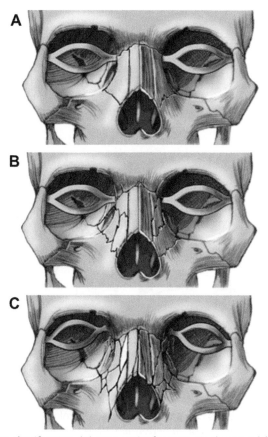

Fig. 5. NOE fracture classification. (*A*) Type I NOE fracture, single central fragment with the medial canthal tendon attached. (*B*) Type II, comminution of the central fragment with the fracture external to the medial canthal tendon-bone insertion. (*C*) Type III, comminution of the central fragment with the medial canthal tendon disrupted from its bony insertion.

nasal septum, and are posteriorly completed through the posterior maxillary walls and pterygoid plates (**Fig. 7**). Le Fort II fractures are known as the pyramidal fracture. They start on one side at the zygomaticomaxillary buttress and cross the face in a superomedial direction leading to a fracture of the inferior orbital rim and orbital floor. They traverse the medial orbit, cross the midline through the nasal bones, and then travel inferolaterally across the contralateral side of the facial skeleton. This causes a pyramidal-shaped inferior facial segment that is separated from the remaining craniofacial skeleton (**Fig. 8**). Similar to Le Fort I, it fractures the nasal septum, the posterior maxillary walls, and the pterygoid plates. Le Fort III fractures cause complete craniofacial separation and occur at the level of the skull base, separating the zygomas from the temporal bones and frontal bones. These fractures cross the lateral medial orbits to reach the midline at the nasofrontal junction. Again, Le Fort III also disrupts the nasal septum and pterygoid plates. Most present day maxillary and complex midfacial fractures are not pure Le Fort fractures, but rather are a combination of the various types.[25] Fracture lines often diverge from the described pathways and may result in mixed-type fractures, unilateral fractures, or other atypical fractures.

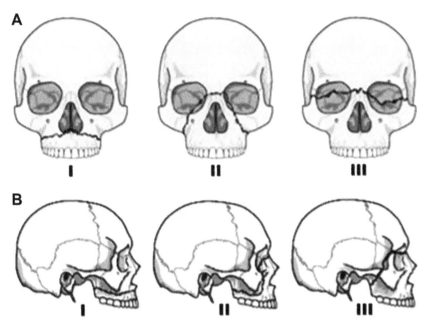

Fig. 6. Classical Le Fort fracture patterns line diagrams (*A*) frontal and (*B*) lateral show the three classic Le Fort fractures. Note that all Le Fort fractures involve the pterygoid plates. (*From* Boeddinghaus R, Whyte A. Current concepts in maxillofacial imaging. Eur J Radiol 2008;66:396–418; with permission.)

PHYSICAL EXAMINATION

Complex midfacial fractures can cause visual and neurologic sequelae. Thus, a thorough physical examination must be performed. Vision should be assessed as soon as possible because progressive visual loss necessitates emergency management. This may be done by shining a light into the eye to assess pupillary response, even in the unresponsive patient. Failure of the pupil to respond may indicate injury to the optic nerve, third cranial nerve, or ciliary ganglion, or a serious intracranial injury. The neurosurgeon and the ophthalmologist must immediately evaluate this condition. Chemosis

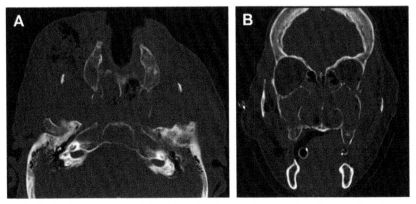

Fig. 7. Le Fort I fracture. (*A*) Axial CT showing the fracture passing through the right pterygoid plate. (*B*) Coronal CT showing the fracture passing through the right and left alveolus.

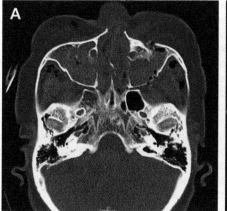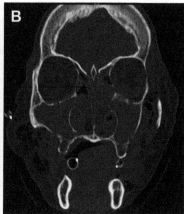

Fig. 8. Le Fort II fracture. (*A*) Axial CT scan indicating a fracture though the left anterior maxillary wall and nasal septum. (*B*) Coronal CT scan for the same patient indicating a fracture though the left zygomaticomaxillary buttress toward the left orbital floor and rim (there is also a right Le Fort I fracture present here).

and subconjunctival hemorrhage, and periorbital ecchymosis are commonly present with zygomatic and orbital injury. Gaze limitation with or without diplopia may also present secondary to extraocular muscle entrapment after midfacial trauma. Forced duction testing and evaluation with applantation tonometer can be performed at the bedside.[26] Globe position should be formally measured or estimated by standing at the head of the bed and comparing eye projection. It should be assessed for enophthalmos versus proptosis (in its anteroposterior position and its vertical position). Enophthalmos may also be identified clinically, either by recognizing the more posterior position of the globe or sometimes by the deepening of the upper lid crease and elongation of the upper lid. If proptosis (from an intraocular hematoma) or orbital apex syndrome (deficit of cranial nerves II, III, IV, V1, or VI) is observed, emergent repair is warranted.[27] Ophthalmologic evaluation should be performed before repair, because some injuries, such as retinal tears, may be a contraindication for surgery. Dependent on the patient's ability to cooperate, a complete cranial nerve examination should also be performed paying close attention to the status of facial nerve function in all regions. If any fluid leakage (otorrhea, rhinorrhea) is seen, it should be studied for possible cerebrospinal fluid leakage and if positive, a neurosurgical consult should be requested.

A patient with ZMC fractures presents with a combination of periorbital and subconjunctival hematoma. Palpation of the zygoma may indicate a deformity; however, this can be obscured if there is a large amount of cheek edema. Paresthesia over the cheek, lateral nose, and upper lips secondary to V2 injury is often present. Ipsilateral epistaxis is common, as is inferior displacement of the zygoma, which may change canthus positioning and subsequently the palpebral fissure. If there is impingement on the coronoid process mandibular motion may also be inhibited.

Ecchymosis and edema localized in the nasal and periorbital regions are associated with isolated NOE fractures; however, NOE and Le Fort fractures that are associated with panfacial fractures are more likely to have diffuse facial edema.[16] Injuries to the NOE complex require careful evaluation of the medial canthal tendon. Injury to the canthal ligament or the bone it attaches to causes displacement of the medial canthal ligament laterally, anteriorly, and inferiorly. This displacement can be missed in the acute setting with soft tissue edema present and may take place gradually. A focused examination should include measurement of the horizontal palpebral widths, the intercanthal distance, and the distance between the nasal dorsal midline and each medial canthus. Average intercanthal distance is 33 to 34 mm for white males and 32 to 34 mm for white females.[24] Intercanthal distances greater than 35 mm suggest that there is displacement of NOE fracture and greater than 40 mm is diagnostic for NOE fracture. A normal examination includes two equal sides and an intercanthal distance that is approximately equal to each horizontal palpebral width, both of which should be equal. Alternative measurements can be done by taking one-half of the interpupillary distance.[28] Reduction of nasal dorsal height and development of epicanthal folds are other physical examination signs commonly seen with NOE fractures.

During evaluation of NOE fracture, direct traction on the medial canthi should be performed to test the firmness of the attachment by pulling it laterally ("bow-string" test). A lack of resistance or movement of the underlying bone indicates a fracture. Paskert and Manson[29] also recommend that a bimanual examination be performed with an instrument, such as a Kelly clamp, in the nose against the medial orbital rim directly opposite the medial canthal ligament and the index finger placed externally, over medial canthal area. In this examination, the examiner tests for stability by assessing movement of the canthus-bearing bone between the Kelly clamp placed against the medial orbital rim and the finger. Movement of the central fragment indicates instability and requires reduction and fixation. If no movement is appreciated operative repair is usually not needed. Thus, the bimanual examination not only helps to confirm the diagnosis of a questionable fracture but it can also determine the need for surgical repair.[16,29]

Le Fort fractures result in interruption of the vertical buttresses and subsequent loss of vertical height of the face. The high force required to induce a Le Fort–type fracture leads to retrusion of the central midface, similar to what is seen in NOE fractures. Fractures leading to displacement or mobility of the maxilla are assessed at the level of the dentition. A change in the patient's occlusion indicates a fracture in either the maxilla or the mandible. Thus, evaluating the teeth first to assess for mobility of their alveolar segments assesses for displacement, which then alters occlusion. If teeth and alveoli are intact mobility of the midface can be assessed by grasping the maxilla at or above the incisors and gently rocking back and forth. This identifies motion relative to either the nasal root or the skull base. Immobility does not guarantee a nonfracture because segments can still be fractured but impacted. One must also assess the hard palate for mucosal tears along the path of the fracture. If the palate is fractured, lingual or buccal projection and significant malposition of the bone fragments may occur.

RADIOLOGIC EVALUATION

Over the past 30 years, high-resolution CT scanning has become the hallmark radiologic modality for assessment of the nature and extent of maxillofacial injuries.[7,30,31] New scanners provide exceptionally fast and accurate results and allow comprehensive coordination of repair of facial fractures in conjunction with injuries to other regions of the body. With the exception of some simple fractures, the CT scan has replaced other forms of radiographic imaging for the assessment of midfacial injuries.

Axial planes are helpful for assessment of the medial and vertical buttresses of the midface and demonstrate changes in the position of the zygomatic arch that may be otherwise missed in high-impact trauma in the coronal direction.[5] They are also helpful for evaluating displacement of maxillary bones and fractures because they travel through the pterygoid plates (Le Fort I and II). If there is also concern for fracture extension into the lateral or medial orbital wall or the optic canal then axial scans should also be evaluated. Imaging of the optic canal and orbital apex takes on critical significance in the presence of cranial neuropathies related to these areas. Visual loss caused by trauma necessitates immediate analysis of orbital CT scans with special attention paid to the lateral orbital rim, because a reversible injury causing constriction of the orbital apex may be identified.[13,14]

Coronal planes are optimal for evaluation of orbital floor blowout fractures and may also be helpful in predicting the amount of enophthalmos that results secondary to orbital wall displacement and the extent of any required repairs.[32–34] Coronal scans are also helpful for nasal bone fractures in combination with injury to the medial orbital wall and frontal process of the maxilla.[25,35] Comminution of the central fragment of the medial orbital wall or loss of bone in the midface may be seen on coronal scans and serves as an indication for bone grafting to reestablish adequate facial projection and restore orbital volume and nasal projection because it precludes reconstruction with plates and screws alone.[24,36] Coronal and parasaggital views are also ideal for evaluation for the optic canal and orbital floor.

TIMING OF TREATMENT

The timing of surgery to repair complex midfacial fractures may vary. Some surgeons prefer to wait for edema to subside before treatment but others argue that it is best to restore bony architecture early. Additionally, in severe trauma stabilization of the patient with life-threatening injuries takes priority. Thus, the level of urgency remains an individual decision.

Orbital and zygomatic fractures can be repaired within 2 to 3 weeks after injury using primary reduction and fixation techniques. Osteotomies may be required after this acute phase up to 4 months after the injury. Delaying care longer may require bone grafting for successful repair.[37] For NOE or Le Fort fractures, the recommendation is to wait no more than 2 weeks.[38] Delayed repair may increase the need for osteotomies to reduce fractures, lead to scarring that interferes with identification of the medial canthal ligament, and prevent adequate correction of intercanthal distance.[16]

TREATMENT GOALS AND PLANNED OUTCOMES
Zygomaticomaxillary Complex Fractures

The degree of injury determines the extent of the surgical exposure needed for repair. If left unrepaired, nondisplaced and minimally displaced fractures may not cause long-term deformity or diplopia.[7] However, severely displaced and comminuted injuries require increased surgical exposure for open reduction and fixation. The goal of ZMC reconstruction is to restore the height, width, and projection of the malar eminence. This is best achieved by reduction with stabilization in three dimensions to maintain the zygoma against the strong masseteric pull. Traditional repairs focused on the most solid fixation point, and it was not uncommon for zygomatic fractures to be repaired with a single wire at the zygomaticofrontal region fracture. However, more recent repair techniques have focused on the zygomaticomaxillary buttress, because this is usually the mobile area, rather than on fixing the zygomaticofrontal hinge point. This lateral buttress is also believed to be an important component of midfacial support, specifically restoring facial height. The surgeon must make several specific decisions, including when to repair; what approaches for exposure to use; which areas to plate; and what type of fixation device (eg, size of titanium plates and screws) to use.

If comminution of the zygomaticomaxillary area occurs, it becomes an inadequate point of reference for reduction. Thus, lower lid exposure may be better to allow for alignment of the infraorbital rim, and for exploration of the orbital floor if needed. Access to the lateral orbit is also particularly helpful, in that alignment of the zygoma with the greater wing of the sphenoid in the lateral orbit tends to be a reliable landmark for bony reduction. Severe comminution of the ZMC may make it even more difficult to be assured that the zygoma has been properly repositioned and a coronal incision allows for full exposure of the entirety of the zygomatic arches. In this case, if the contralateral zygoma is intact, it may serve as a good frame of reference. Finally, alterations in occlusion may require intermaxillary fixation before fracture reduction. Evaluation of the class of occlusion before surgery is a critical step that should not be ignored.

Each ZMC fracture should be reduced and fixated with the goal of using the least amount of plating and disruption of soft tissue.[39] This may be achieved with miniplate-and-screw fixation at the zygomaticomaxillary buttresses, zygomaticofrontal suture, inferior orbital rim, or the zygomatic arch. It is not always necessary to plate each of these fracture sites. Variable sizes of plates are available (1–2 mm). Plating is best performed under wide exposure for accurate placement and fixation of the arch. Although large plates can be used to reestablish the shape of the lateral face and provide strength to overcome masseteric pull, smaller plates or bioresorbable plating at the zygomaticofrontal and infraorbital rim are helpful to avoid patient complaints of feeling the plates postoperatively. Studies of these bioresorbable plating systems alone, or in combination with titanium, indicate that there is no difference in postoperative bone stability and they were sufficiently strong to overcome masseteric forces.[3,40]

Several approaches for repair of ZMC fractures are available including the subciliary or transconjunctival incision, a lateral brow or upper blepharoplasty incision, a gingival buccal incision, and the coronal or hemicoronal incision. External lacerations may also assist with exposure to the facial skeleton.[38] The zygomaticofrontal suture can be fixated through an extended upper blepharoplasty incision or by the coronal approach. Fixation of the infraorbital rim can be done through a subciliary or transconjunctival incision that allows for accurate placement of bony fragments and for the exposure to place prosthetic material to reconstruct the orbital floor. Recent data support transconjunctival incisions and lateral cantholysis to avoid visible scarring and potential complications.[41,42] The zygomaticofrontal suture may also be accessed through this incision. Zygomaticomaxillary buttresses are exposed through a gingivobuccal incision; however, this approach does place the infraorbital nerve at risk. Bone grafting may be necessary for additional support at the lateral or medial buttress. This is performed in cases of severe communition, in which there is inadequate bone to plate.

If lateral displacement and severe comminution are present and the entirety of the zygomatic arch must be visualized, a coronal or hemicoronal approach is indicated. The coronal approach may also be used for accurate reduction and fixation of the arch to the temporal bone. With this approach, care must be taken to avoid injuring the frontal branch of the facial nerve within the temporoparietal fascia and the temporal fat pad, which is prone to atrophy and subsequent temporal wasting on injury. With coronal dissection, the supraorbital nerve may also be reduced if necessary from its notch to gain access to bony fragments.

Orbital Fractures

Indications for surgical repair of orbital fractures are controversial but strong indications for surgery include enopthalmos greater than 2 mm, significant hypoglobus, or diplopia.[43] Most patients with orbital fractures are first evaluated by ophthalmology to rule out visual loss. If vision is stable, three critical findings are evaluated to assess for the need for repair: (1) entrapment of extraocular muscles without ocular mobility, (2) herniation of greater than 50% of orbital contents into the maxillary sinus with impending globe malposition, and (3) optic canal injury. The latter may be presupposed if the orbital apex and middle cranial fossa are impacted by high force to the lateral orbital wall and impinge on the apex.[5]

A recent literature review demonstrates that use of the transconjunctival approach to access the orbit is continually increasing.[44] The transconjunctival incision offers excellent visualization and is associated with a reduced risk of ectropion and permanent scleral show compared with the subciliary approach.[45–47] However, for placement of large grafts and exposure of the medial and lateral orbits it does require the addition of the lateral canthotomy. This does have the potential for a higher incidence of entropion and displacement of the lateral canthus so care must be taken with reapproximation.[46,48] In the case of older patients with pronounced wrinkling and lower lid laxity, the subciliary incision may be an option that offers access to the infraorbital rim with a minimal risk of retraction.[48,49]

The medial orbit can be explored by a transconjunctival incision, coronal incision, or cutaneous incision similar to an external ethmoidectomy approach. If a lower lid incision is used, a Frost stitch must also be placed temporarily to stretch the lower lid and decrease the likelihood of lower lid malposition. However, the advent of the transconjunctival incision has all but eliminated the need for the Frost suture to suspend the lower eyelid from the forehead during early healing.[50] The lateral orbital rim was commonly accessed through the lateral brow incision. However, because of the presence of a noticeable scar, the upper lid blepharoplasty incision has become increasingly popular because it can be easily hidden in the upper lid crease.[5] The lateral rim can also be reached through a transconjunctival incision, when the incision is extended laterally and a canthotomy is performed.

The first step in management of orbital fractures is to restore the orbit to its preinjury shape. This requires a familiarity with the normal orbital contours. Assistance may be found in a model skull to help with prebending implants that can be sterilized for use during the procedure. It is also important to recognize the convexity on the orbital floor medially behind the equator of the globe and in the medial wall because inadequate reconstitution affects globe position.[5] Finally, forced duction testing should be performed after all trapped orbital tissues (fat/muscle) are released from fractures.

Alloplastic (resorbable and nonresorbable) and autologous materials can be used to reconstruct the orbital wall contours. Reconstruction of a defect of the concave anterior floor can usually be adequately accomplished with an alloplastic implant with close attention paid to completely exposing two opposing quadrants of the defect for stable support of the implant.[50] During repair the surgeon must take into account that the distance from the edge of the floor to apex is approximately 4.5 to 5 cm to prevent using an implant that is too large and compresses the apex.

Porous polyethylene is an ideal choice for repair of orbital floor defects because it is easily available, can easily be bent or trimmed, and does not necessarily require fixation.[50,51] The use of low-profile (1–1.3 mm) titanium plates or mesh is helpful because they are thin, stiff, easy to contour, and can be easily stabilized. In addition, they have the unique ability to compensate for volume without the potential for resorption. Recently, the use of titanium mesh has come under some scrutiny.[52–55] Lee and Nunery[55] associated these implants with adherence of orbital and periorbital structures resulting in restrictive diplopia or eyelid retraction. Thus, one should closely monitor patients for early signs of adherence syndrome because an intense fibrotic adherence may occur between the titanium implant within the orbit or periorbital tissues making it extremely difficult to remove. Split calvarial bone is also readily available and easily harvested. It is suited for reconstruction of larger defects, such as the concave anterior and convex posterior floor that require greater rigidity.[50] Split rib can also be used, because it is more pliable than bone and can be molded to shape, but it does undergo greater resorption.[5]

NOE Fractures

NOE fractures are among the most difficult to repair and various surgical approaches have been considered. Wide access and wide exposure provide the best opportunity for a good outcome. Thus, the coronal incision remains the gold standard for access to the nasofrontal suture region and to the medial orbital walls. This incision also allows access to the parietal bone for harvesting dorsal strut graft. Other approaches include the Lynch incision and midfacial degloving, which avoids a facial or scalp incision, but leads to difficulty gaining access to the orbital floor and medial orbital wall.[56] In conjunction with the coronal incision, the transconjunctival or subciliary incisions may also be helpful for accessing the inferior orbital rim and orbital floor in NOE repair. Additionally, the maxillary vestibular incision may also be helpful to gain access to the piriform rim if necessary.

The goal of the surgeon is to reconstruct the disrupted medial canthal tendon to adequately withstand the constant lateral tension of the lids. Otherwise, telecanthus is likely, and poor function of the lacrimal collecting system may result. Type I injuries, where the medial canthal ligaments remain attached to a large fragment of bone, are the most simple to repair (see **Fig. 5**A). This is done by stabilizing the bone to the surrounding skeleton with plates (1–1.3 mm). Three-point stabalization is recommended using rigid fixation at the nasofrontal junction, infraorbital rim, and piriform rim.[57] If not properly fixed, it may lateralize and lead to significant deformity over time. Repair of the more severe type II and III injuries is controversial (see **Fig. 5**B, C). Some authors believe the surgeon should preserve any of the ligamentous attachments to bone, whereas others advocate focusing on the ligaments alone.[58–61] For type II and III injuries, fixation of the bony fragments can be performed with a combination of microplates for larger bony segments and wires for smaller segments. Typically 28- or 30-gauge wires are used. An overcorrection result is preferred to an undercorrected telecanthus.[5]

Identification of the medial canthal tendon may be difficult. If it is avulsed from the bone, grasping tissue in the region of the tendon and pulling medially may help to locate it. After the medial canthal tendon is located, a 28- or 30-gauge wire is passed through the bony fragment for the transnasal canthopexy. If there is severe comminution and the wire cannot be secured through the fragments, a permanent suture may then be secured through the tendon and the other end of the suture is secured to a wire. The wire is then passed through the nasal bones using a spinal needle to perform the transnasal canthopexy.[57] The wire is passed through the ligament and is passed through the area of the posterior lacrimal crest, posterior to the nasal bones, through the nasal septum, and out the contralateral side. One must be certain to avoid injury to the contralateral globe, which should be protected with a malleable retractor. At this time the wire may be fixed to the contralateral frontal bone through a plate hole, a hole in the supraorbital rim, or to the contralateral medial canthal ligament. Tightening the wire then fixes medial canthal ligaments together reducing the intercanthal distance. No lateral flaring should be present at the posterior aspect of the fracture because if the ligament is not fixed medially, it lateralizes over time and results in telecanthus, malposition of the caruncle, horizontal shortening of the lids, and potential lacrimal dysfunction.[5,57]

With type II and III injuries reconstruction of the nasal dorsum must also be performed to reestablish nasal projection. Failure to do so tends to exaggerate any appearance of telecanthus and increases the likelihood of developing epicanthal folds. This may be done with calvarial bone harvest or with rib, iliac crest, mandible, or cadaveric irradiated rib. This is necessary for many reasons including the loss of support from a weakened septum, comminution of bones in the area, and prevention of a saddle nose.[16,36,38,58,59] In type III fractures, the medial orbital wall may also require reconstruction with a bone graft to provide a stable strut of bone for reattachment of the medial canthal tendon and to prevent enopthalmos.[16,36]

Le Fort Fractures

For treatment of Le Fort–type fractures, the surgical access required depends greatly on the fracture pattern. Le Fort I fractures may be accessed by a gingivobuccal sulcus incision.[60] Incising the mucosa of the gingivobuccal sulcus provides access to the anterior maxillary walls, including the piriform apertures, the frontal processes, and the zygomaticomaxillary junction. This incision allows elevation superiorly to the infraorbital rims. The midfacial degloving approach may also be used; however, this does add the risk of nasal stenosis because the mucosa of the nasal vestibule is incised circumferentially.[5]

Primary stabilization of Le Fort and other midfacial fractures that involve tooth-bearing segments should be performed at the level of the occlusion. Le Fort I fractures above the occlusal level are repaired by reestablishing the midfacial buttresses using 1.5- to 2-mm L and J plates. To prevent the forces of mastication from disrupting the repair, emphasis must be put on placing these in the same direction as the forces of mastication.[61] If the palate is fractured and severe disruption occurs at the alveolar segments or the mandible, a palatal splint may be needed to correct dentition. The palate may be repaired directly with a plate, or it may be stabilized along the premaxillary area if the occlusal stabilization is adequate to prevent rotation.

Le Fort II and III fractures may require a coronal incision with additional exposure by the transconjunctival, subciliary, or lateral brow incisions.[60] These are best stabilized also by using 1.5- to 2-mm L and J plates and the infraorbital rim may be plated to stabilize the superior level of the fractures. Additionally, the maxilla must be disimpacted, mandibulomaxillary fixation (MMF) should be implemented, and the nasal root should be rigidly fixated for Le Fort II and III fractures. The buttresses are very important for structural support. Similar to NOE fracture repair, if bone is deficient along these buttresses, it should be replaced with split calvarium and stabilized under a plate, or it may be used as a biologic plate and fixed to the bone at each end using lag screws. A defect less than 5 mm in a single buttress can be safely bridged with a plate; however, if the defect is larger it should be bridged using bone grafts from another site.[5,62]

COMPLICATIONS OF SURGERY FOR MIDFACIAL TRAUMA

Failure to achieve ideal reduction is the most common complication from management of midfacial trauma. When the bone heals in the incorrect position, a malunion results. In the face, this leads to asymmetry. If the zygoma, orbit, and globe are involved, such malpositions as enophthalmos with subsequent diplopia may result. If the orbital floor has been inadequately reconstituted hypophthalmos may also be seen. Failure to adequately repair the position of the medial canthal tendon leads to telecanthus. If proper occlusion is not addressed before midfacial fracture reduction and fixation, a malocclusion results. These deformities may require reexploration and placement of additional graft material.[5,57]

In addition to management of the bony segments, soft tissue management is critical. With elevation of the midface, the periosteum may be stripped when accessing the lateral or medial buttresses. Ectropion is a relatively frequent complication of midfacial fracture repairs, particularly when the orbital floor is explored, or the inferior orbital rim is plated. Meticulous technique, the avoidance of titanium when possible, and resuspension of the midfacial soft tissues can all help prevent this. Fixation can occur by a suture ligature around the periosteum or around a plate screw to prevent downward pull and potential ectropion. Suture fixation of the nasal alae subcutaneously may also prevent alar base widening after use of the midface degloving approach. Branches of the trigeminal and facial nerve are at risk during multiple facial exposures, and great care should be exercised to avoid injuring these important structures.

Extreme care must also be exercised when exploring the orbit. Hematoma after orbital floor repair may lead to permanent visual loss and patients should be admitted for serial postoperative visual checks. The lacrimal collecting system can also be injured during surgery and if its continuity is in question, cannulation of the canaliculi and stenting are recommended. Injury to the extraocular muscles and their nerves can result in diplopia, even in the absence of entrapment.

POSTPROCEDURAL CARE

Postoperative antibiotics may be given for 5 to 10 days depending on the exposure of fracture sites to the external environment or communication with intraoral or intranasal spaces. Coverage should be against gram-positive and anaerobic organisms. For any fracture requiring restoration of the orbital floor the authors observe patients overnight with serial visual examinations. If wire fixation was used for MMF, wire cutters should be placed near the patient at all times in the early postoperative period to allow the patient to expel vomited material and wires or rubber bands should be removed if the patient begins to feel nauseated.

After discharge patients should be evaluated within 1 week for suture removal and evaluation for the wounds. Follow-up should continue at 2 to 4 weeks, and additionally at 3 to 8 weeks if removal of MMF is needed. Depending on the severity of the deformity longer-term follow-up care may be needed. For patients in MMF it is essential to keep patients in a state of facial immobilization. This period may range from 4 to 8 weeks. This requires that MMF be maintained during this period and requires good oral hygiene by the patient. For Le Fort–type fractures, it is important to test the stability of the repair by palpating the facial skeleton along the patient's maxillary teeth during clenching and relaxing of the muscles of mastication. Minimal motion is acceptable, but excessive mobility may indicate poor healing. Postoperative imaging should be performed in patients in whom malunion is suggested. Excess motion along the vertical buttresses is also a contraindication to removing the arch bars. After the facial bones are healed and normal occlusion is present, the MMF may be removed.

FUTURE ADVANCEMENTS
Minimal Access Endoscopic-assisted Techniques for Facial Trauma

The goal of the endoscopic approach for facial trauma repair is to perform stable anatomic reduction while taking maximal advantage of minimal access approaches. Taking advantage of long lever arms and magnification capabilities of endoscopic instruments permits surgeons to work through small stab incisions, protecting important structures and decreasing the need for wide soft tissue degloving.[63] Several studies have evaluated endoscopic approaches for complex zygoma fractures, orbital floor and blowout fractures, and Le Fort III injuries. There have been no reported cases of permanent palsy, orbital hemorrhage, or optic nerve, ocular globe, or extraocular muscle injury; however, extended operative times, temporary facial nerve palsy, and injury to the nasolacrimal duct have been reported.[64–67] As experience with endoscopic approaches improves, the morbidity of surgical access will further decrease in the treatment of complex midface fractures where open reduction and internal fixation was once considered standard.

SUMMARY

The midfacial skeleton is composed of vertical and horizontal buttresses that support function and protect vital organs. High-impact injury to the midface causes complex fracture patterns. Diagnosis and treatment requires a thorough understanding of the facial skeleton and appreciation for cosmetic and functional deformity. The goal of treatment is to restore the bony infrastructure while disrupting the least amount of soft tissue. Treatment has evolved from wide field exposure techniques to smaller, well-concealed incisions and miniplate fixation. Future developments and improvement of endoscopic techniques may further decrease the morbidity of surgical access for complex midfacial trauma.

REFERENCES

1. Manson PN, Hoops JE, Su CT. Structural pillars of the facial skeleton: an approach to the management of Le Fort fractures. Plast Reconstr Surg 1980; 66(1):54–62.
2. Stanley RB. Reconstruction of the midface vertical dimension following Le Fort fractures. Arch Otorhinolaryngol 1984;110(9):571–5.
3. Karlan MS, Cassissi NJ. Fractures of the zygoma, a geometric, biomechanical, and surgical analysis. Arch Otorhinolaryngol 1979;105(6):320–7.
4. Perry M. Maxillofacial trauma – developments, innovations and controversies. Injury 2008;40(12):1252–9.
5. Kellman RM. Maxillofacial trauma. In: Flint PW, editor. Cumming's otolaryngology, head & neck surgery, vol. 23, 5th edition. Philadelphia: Mosby; 2010. p. 318–41.
6. Evans BG, Evans GR. Zygomatic fractures. Plast Reconstr Surg 2008;121(Suppl 1): 1–11.
7. Manson PN, Markowitz B, Mirvis S, et al. Toward CT-based facial fracture treatment. Plast Reconstr Surg 1990;85(2):202–12.
8. Zingg M, Laedrach K, Chen J, et al. Classification and treatment of zygomatic fractures: a review of 1,025 cases. J Oral Maxillofac Surg 1992;50(8):778–90.
9. Ellis E, El-Attar A, Moos FK. An analysis of 2,067 cases of zygomatic orbital fracture. J Oral Maxillofac Surg 1985;43(6):417–28.
10. Pearl RM. Treatment of enopthalmos. Clin Plast Surg 1992;19(1):99–111.
11. Markowitz BL, Manson PN. Panfacial fractures: organization of treatment. Clin Plast Surg 1989;16(1):105–14.
12. Stack BC, Ruggiero FP. Maxillary and periorbital fractures. In: Bailey BJ, Johnson JT, Newlands S, editors. Head & neck surgery – otolaryngology, vol. 1, 4th edition. Philadelphia: Lippincott Williams, Wilkins; 2006. p. 975–93.
13. Funk GF, Stanley RB, Becker TS. Reversible visual loss due to impacted lateral orbital wall fractures. Head Neck Surg 1989;11(4):295–300.

14. Stanley RB. The temporal approach to impacted lateral orbital wall fractures. Arch Otolaryngol Head Neck Surg 1988;114(4):550–3.
15. Shelton D. Nasal-orbital-ethmoid fractures. In: Alling CI, Osbon D, editors. Maxillofacial trauma. Philadelphia: Lea & Febiger; 1988. p. 363–71.
16. Leipziger LS, Manson PN. Nasoethmoid orbital fractures. Current concepts and management principles. Clin Plast Surg 1992;19(1):167–93.
17. Blair VP, Brown JB, Hamm WG. Surgery of the inner canthus and related structures. Am J Ophthalmol 1932;15:498.
18. Converse JM, Smith B. Canthoplasty and dacrocystorhinostomy in malunited fractures of the medial wall of the orbit. Am J Ophthalmol 1952;35(8):1103–14.
19. Converse JM, Smith B. Naso-orbital fractures. Trans Am Acad Ophthalmol Otolaryngol 1963;67:622–34.
20. Converse JM, Smith B. Naso-orbital fractures and traumatic deformities of the medial canthus. Plast Reconstr Surg 1966;38(2):147–62.
21. Holt GR, Holt JE. Nasoethmoid complex injuries. Otolaryngol Clin North Am 1985;18(1):87–8.
22. Gruss JS. Fronto-naso-orbital trauma. Clin Plast Surg 1982;9(4):577–89.
23. Becelli R, Renzi G, Mannino G. Postraumatic obstruction of lacrimal pathways: a retrospective analysis of 58 consecutive naso-orbitoethmoid fractures. J Craniofac Surg 2004;15(1):29–33.
24. Markowitz BL, Manson PN, Sargent L, et al. Management of the medial canthal tendon in nasoethmoid fractures: the importance of the central fragment in classification and treatment. Plast Reconstr Surg 1991;87(5):843–53.
25. Fraioli RE, Branstetter BF, Deleyiannis FW. Facial fractures: beyond Le Fort. Otolaryngol Clin North Am 2008;41(1):51–76.
26. Kellman RM, Bersani T. Delayed and secondary repair of posttraumatic enophthalmos and orbital deformities. Facial Plast Surg Clin North Am 2002;10(3):311–23.
27. Stanley RB. The zygomatic arch as a guide to reconstruction of comminuted malar fractures. Arch Otolaryngol Head Neck Surg 1989;115(12):1459–62.
28. Holt JE, Holt GR. Ocular and orbital trauma. Washington, DC: American Academy of Otolaryngology-Head and Neck Surgery Foundation, Inc.; 1983.
29. Paskert JP, Manson PN. Nasoethmoid and orbital fractures. Clin Plast Surg 1988;15(2):209–23.
30. Besenski N. Traumatic injuries: imaging of head injuries. Eur Radiol 2002;12(6):1237–52.
31. Russel J, Davidson M, Daly B, et al. Computed tomography in the diagnosis of maxillofacial trauma. Br J Oral Maxillofac Surg 1990;28(5):287–91.
32. Manson PN, Grivas A, Rosenbaum A, et al. Studies on enophthalmos. II. The measurement of orbital injuries and their treatment by quantitative computed tomography. Plast Reconstr Surg 1986;77(2):203–14.
33. Parsons GS, Mathog RH. Orbital wall and volume relationships. Arch Otolaryngol Head Neck Surg 1988;114(7):743–7.
34. Rubin PA, Bilyk JR, Shore JW. Management of orbital trauma: fractures, hemorrhage, and traumatic optic neuropathy. Focal Points Amer Acad Ophthalmology 1994;12:1.
35. Hopper RA, Salemy S, Sze RW. Diagnosis of midface fractures with CT: what the surgeon needs to know. Radiographics 2006;26(3):783–93.
36. Herford AS, Ying T, Brown B. Outcomes of severely comminuted (type III) nasoorbitoethmoid fractures. J Oral Maxillofac Surg 2005;63(9):1266–77.
37. Carr RM, Mathog RH. Early and delayed repair of orbitozygomatic complex fractures. J Oral Maxillofac Surg 1997;55(3):253–8.

38. Ellis E. Sequencing treatment for naso-orbito-ethmoid fractures. J Oral Maxillofac Surg 1993;51(5):543–58.
39. Meslemani D, Kellman RM. Zygomaticomaxillary complex fractures. Arch Facial Plast Surg 2012;14(1):62–6.
40. Hanemann M, Simmon O, Jain S, et al. A comparison of combinations of titanium and resorbable plating systems for repair of isolated zygomatic fractures in the adult: a quantitative biomechanical study. Ann Plast Surg 2005;54(4): 402–8.
41. Hozle F, Swaid S, Schiwy T, et al. Management of zygomatic fractures via a transconjunctival approach with lateral canthotomy while preserving the lateral ligament. Mund Kiefer Gesichtschir 2004;8(5):296–301 [in German].
42. Zhong LP, Chen GF. Subciliary incision and lateral canthotolysis in rigid internal fixation of zygomatic complex fractures. Chin J Traumatol 2004;7(3):170–4.
43. Kontio R, Lindqvist C. Management of orbital fractures. Oral Maxillofac Surg Clin North Am 2009;21(2):209–20.
44. Gosau M, Schöneich M, Draenert FG, et al. Retrospective analysis of orbital floor fractures—complications, outcome, and review of literature. Clin Oral Investig 2011;15(3):305–13.
45. Ben Simon GJ, Molina M, Schwarcz RM, et al. External (subciliary) vs internal (transconjunctival) involutional entropion repair. Am J Ophthalmol 2005;139(3): 482–7.
46. De Riu G, Meloni SM, Gobbi R, et al. Subciliary versus swinging eyelid approach to the orbital floor. J Craniomaxillofac Surg 2008;36(8):439–42.
47. Appling WD, Patrinely JR, Salzer TA. Transconjunctival approach vs subciliary skin-muscle flap approach for orbital fracture repair. Arch Otolaryngol Head Neck Surg 1993;119(9):1000–7.
48. Cole P, Boyd V, Banerji S, et al. Comprehensive management of orbital fractures. Plast Reconstr Surg 2007;120(7 Suppl 2):57–63.
49. Bähr W, Bagambis FB, Schlegel G, et al. Comparison of transcutaneous incisions used for exposure of the infraorbital rim. Plast Reconstr Surg 1992; 90(4):585–91.
50. Ishii LI, Byrne PJ, Stanley RB. Orbitozygomatic fractures. In: Papel I, editor. Facial plastic and reconstructive surgery. 3rd edition. New York: Thieme; 2002. p. 965–75.
51. Wellisz T. Clinical experience with medpor porous polyethylene acid implant. Aesthetic Plast Surg 1993;17(4):339–44.
52. Ellis E, Tan Y. Assessment of internal orbitl reconstruction for pure blowout fractures: cranial bone grafts versus titanium mesh. J Oral maxillofac Surg 2003; 61(4):442–53.
53. Sugar AW, Kuriakose M, Walshaw ND. Titanium mesh in orbital wall reconstruction. Int J Oral Maxillofac Surg 1992;21(3):140–4.
54. Mackenzie DJ, Arora B, Hansen J. Orbital floor repair with titanium mesh scree. J Craniomaxillofac Trauma 1999;5(3):9–16.
55. Lee HB, Nunery WR. Orbital adherence syndrome secondary to titanium implant material. Ophthal Plast Reconstr Surg 2009;25(1):33–6.
56. Cultura A, Turk JB, Gady HE. Midfacial degloving approach for repair of naso-orbital-ethmoid and midfacial fractures. Arch Facial Plast Surg 2004;6(2):133–5.
57. Papadopoulous H, Salib NK. Management of naso-orbito-ethmoidal fractures. Oral Maxillofac Surg Clin North Am 2009;21(2):221–5.
58. Gruss JS, MacKinnon SE, Kassel EE, et al. The role of primary bone grafting in complex craniomaxillofacial trauma. Plast Reconstr Surg 1985;75(1):17–24.

59. Gruss JS. Complex nasoethmoid-orbital and midfacial fractures: role of cranio-facial surgical techniques and immediate bone grafting. Ann Plast Surg 1986; 17(5):377–90.

60. Manson PN. Management of midfacial fractures. In: Georgiade G, Georgiade N, Riefkohl R, editors. Textbook of plastic, maxillofacial and reconstructive surgery, vol. 1, 2nd edition. Baltimore (MD): William & Wilkins; 1992. p. 409–32.

61. Rudderman RH, Mullen RL. Biomechanics of the facial skeleton. Clin Plast Surg 1992;19(1):11–29.

62. Kellman RM, Marentette LJ. Atlas of craniomaxillofacial fixation. New York: Raven Press; 1995.

63. Lee C, Czerwinski M. Applications of the endoscope in facial fracture manage-ment. Semin Plast Surg 2008;22(1):29–36.

64. Lee CH, Lee C, Trabulsy PP, et al. A cadaveric and clinical evaluation of endo-scopically assisted zygomatic fracture repair. Plast Reconstr Surg 1998;101(2): 333–45.

65. Chen CT, Lai JP, Chen YR. Application of endoscope in zygomatic fracture repair. Br J Plast Surg 2000;53(2):100–5.

66. Strong EB. Endoscopic repair of orbital blow-out fractures. Facial Plast Surg 2004;20(3):223–30.

67. Chen CT, Chen YR. Endoscopically assisted repair of orbital floor fractures. Plast Reconstr Surg 2001;108(7):2011–8.

Condylar Fractures

Raja Sawhney, MD, MFA[a], Ryan Brown, MD[b],
Yadranko Ducic, MD, FRCS(C)[c,d],*

KEYWORDS

- Condylar fractures • Mandible fractures • Endoscopic fracture repair

KEY POINTS

- There is a role for both open and closed reduction in the treatment of condylar fractures.
- Using a thoughtful approach with an understanding of the pros and cons of each treatment option, applied individually to each patient fracture, leads to the best long-term outcomes while minimizing the sequelae associated with surgery.
- Careful unbiased critique of postoperative results with the goal of continually improving techniques and outcomes is, in the end, significantly beneficial to both patients and surgeons.

OVERVIEW

No area of facial trauma elicits as much debate as the treatment of fractures of the condylar region. Optimal treatment seems to vary as much by surgical subspecialty as by treating surgeons themselves. Some of this variability is derived from surgeon comfort with different surgical techniques and approaches as well as concern for vital surrounding structures.[1] Earlier publications on the treatment of these types of fractures attempted to determine whether open or closed treatment is the optimal choice.[2] Recent discussions have shifted, with the understanding that both treatments have their indications. What is open for debate is when each option should be used.

Condylar fractures account for 20% to 62% of all mandibular fractures.[3] Traditionally, closed management has been the most advocated treatment. As new techniques were developed and a better understanding of the associated sequelae of closed reduction elicited, there was a trend toward more surgical reduction of the fracture. Rigid rules with fairly wide indications for the implementation of open approaches were proposed, but concerns arose regarding whether these rules were leading to

[a] Department of Otolaryngology–Head and Neck Surgery, University of Florida, 200 Southwest 62nd Boulevard, Suite B, Gainesville, FL 32607, USA; [b] Department of Head and Neck Surgery, Kaiser Permanente, 2045 Franklin Street, Denver, CO 80205, USA; [c] Department of Otolaryngology–Head and Neck Surgery, University of Texas Southwestern Medical Center, Dallas, TX, USA; [d] Otolaryngology and Facial Plastic Surgery Associates, 923 Pennsylvania Avenue, Suite 100, Fort Worth, TX 76104, USA
* Corresponding author. Otolaryngology and Facial Plastic Surgery Associates, 923 Pennsylvania Avenue, Suite 100, Fort Worth, TX 76104.
E-mail address: yducic@sbcglobal.net

Otolaryngol Clin N Am 46 (2013) 779–790
http://dx.doi.org/10.1016/j.otc.2013.06.003   oto.theclinics.com

unnecessary surgery, with increases in morbidity, surgical time, and risk to the facial nerve. A middle ground has developed, where there is an understanding of those patients who can be treated successfully with simple closed reduction and those better served with open reduction of their condylar fracture.

There are few absolute indications for the open treatment of condylar fracture. If adequate occlusion cannot be obtained through closed reduction, then open reduction is necessary. Most agree that condylar fractures in conjunction with significant comminuted midface fractures warrants condylar reduction. In difficult midface fractures, the intact mandible is used as a stable base from which to reset maxillary dentition, re-establish occlusion, and then rebuild the midface as a whole, in a bottom to top fashion.[4] By recreating appropriate occlusion, proper maxillary projection and width can be re-established.

Ellis and colleagues[4] maintain the need for open treatment in edentulous patients and in those missing significant posterior dentition. In these cases, closed reduction cannot adequately address the loss of vertical mandibular height that is normally re-established when appropriate posterior dentition is present. This loss of height leads to altered jaw mechanics with significant deviation toward the fractured side or, in the case of bilateral fractures, open bite deformity. The derived malocclusion is difficult to treat later with prosthesis. Bilateral condylar fractures is an area where treatment is more controversial. Ellis has found that 10% of patients in this cohort do not respond well to closed treatment. Unfortunately, which patients are recalcitrant to closed treatment is unclear. Some investigators have argued that significantly severe dislocation of the fractured condyle is an indication for open reduction and internal fixation.[5] Studies have shown this not to be the case and that, through remodeling, appropriate occlusion can be re-established despite the visible alteration in jaw mechanics.[4]

TREATMENT GOALS AND PLANNED OUTCOMES

The principal goal of treatment is re-establishment of normal occlusion and mastication.[1] Beyond this, restoration of baseline jaw mechanics and overall cosmesis are also given consideration. As discussed previously, the ideal surgical technique to obtain these goals is variable and based on individual injury while weighing the risk/benefit of surgery.

PREOPERATIVE PLANNING AND PREPARATION

As with any other surgery, patient safety is of penultimate importance. Patient stability before surgery must be assessed with associated preoperative evaluation and laboratory work. Comorbid injuries are not unusual and need to be assessed in regards to urgency and triage of treatment. A surgical plan must be determined. Patients require adequate dentition or at least intact dentures to even consider closed reduction or mandibular–maxillary fixation. If endoscopic reduction is planned, appropriate equipment is necessary that may not be readily available.[6] With external approaches, obtaining cervical spine clearance and removal of cervical collar allows the head to be turned, making surgery significantly easier.

PATIENT POSITIONING

With either an open or closed approach, it is likely patients are placed in maxillary–mandibular fixation, if only intraoperatively. Therefore, nasotracheal intubation is used in most cases, with the circuit brought up over the head and secured with a head wrap. In cases where this is not a possibility, due to comorbid injuries or need for long-term ventilator support, then a tracheostomy must be considered. Regardless of treatment planned, the arms are tucked and the table is turned 180° to allow several surgeons and assistants access to the head.

PROCEDURAL APPROACHES
Pediatric Condylar Fractures

Condylar fractures are the most common pediatric mandibular fracture and present bilaterally in 20% of cases.[7] Prior to age 6, most fractures are intracapsular, whereas after that age they occur most frequently in the neck of the mandible. When normal occlusion is present, fractures of the condylar region are treated conservatively with close observation, soft diet, and pain medication. When there is malocclusion, a short course of maxillary–mandibular fixation is warranted. Limiting fixation to 7 to 10 days helps limit the chance of joint ankylosis, although postoperative physiotherapy may still be beneficial. Choice of technique is largely dependent on the age of the child and, more importantly, the quality and quantity of dentition. When possible, intradental wires with arch bars maybe placed. If not possible, intermaxillary fixation using 1-point circumandibular wiring should be used, attaching it to a wire wrapped around a hole drilled through piriform aperture. Due to the possibility of injuring nonerupted teeth, intermaxillary fixation screws should not be placed. It is important to discuss chin deviation during chewing and the possibility of long-term growth abnormalities of the jaw with patients' parents.

Closed Reduction

Several approaches for closed reduction may be used. The authors have found that obtaining occlusion with elastic bands offers the same benefit as metal wiring but permits patients to subtly shift into natural occlusion while mobilizing earlier, which improves dietary intake and lowers the chance of joint ankylosis. If there are concerns about patient compliance with elastics, surgeons may elect to stay with the reliability of complete wire fixation.

Preauricular Approach

The preauricular approach is excellent to expose the temporomandibular joint (TMJ) and to remove displaced condylar fragments. The incision also hides well in the pre-auricular crease. It provides, however, poor exposure and visualization of the sub-condylar region. If placing a fixation plate and screws is desired, it often requires inferior retraction on the facial nerve, potentially causing paresis (**Fig. 1**).

The incision is marked in a skin crease in front of the pinna beginning at the superior pole of the helix and extending inferiorly to the inferior anterior edge of the tragus. The incision is carried through skin and subcutaneous tissues. Superior to the zygomatic arch, the temporoparietal fascia is incised to reach the superficial layer of the deep temporal fascia, with care taken to avoid damaging the superficial temporal vessels and auriculotemporal nerve. Inferior to the zygomatic arch, the dissection precedes to the same depth as the superior dissection, immediately anterior to the tragal carti-lage. In the superior portion of the incision, the superficial layer of the deep temporal fascia is then incised starting at the anterior superior portion of the incision and running at a 30° angle to the long axis of the helix, toward the tragus. This exposes a layer of fat between the superficial and deep layers of the deep temporal fascia, and a periosteal elevator can be inserted in this incision deep to the superficial layer of the deep temporal fascia. The periosteal elevator can be used to free the periosteum off of the lateral zygomatic arch and create a tunnel inferior to the zygomatic arch. The

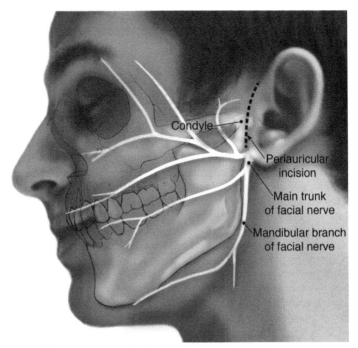

Fig. 1. The dashed line represents the incision for the preauricular approach. The relationship between the incision, the condyle, and the facial nerve is seen.

intervening tissue can then sharply be divided posteriorly along the original axis of the vertical skin incision. This subperiosteal flap can then be reflected anteriorly from the root of the zygomatic arch, thus protecting the temporal branch of the facial nerve. Dissection proceeds anteriorly until the articular eminence and entire TMJ capsule should be revealed. To help locate and palpate this, the mandible can be opened and closed. Dissection and retraction can proceed inferiorly to reveal the subcondylar region.[8–11]

Submandibular/Risdon Approach

The submandibular/Risdon approach provides good access to the ramus and lower subcondylar areas of the mandible but can be somewhat limited for high subcondylar or condylar fractures because the incision is positioned a long ways away from these fractures. The main complication is either paralysis or paresis of the marginal mandibular branch of the facial nerve either from direct injury or from retraction forces. The scar created is also visible on the neck.

The 4-cm to 5-cm incision is marked 1 to 2 fingerbreadths below the inferior border of the mandible near the angle (**Fig. 2**). Care should be taken to hide the incision within a skin crease if possible. The dissection proceeds through skin and subcutaneous tissue until the superoinferiorly oriented fibers of the platysma muscle are identified. The platysma is divided to reveal the superficial layer of the deep cervical fascia, the submandibular gland in the anterior aspect of the incision, and often the facial artery and vein. The marginal mandibular branch of the facial nerve is located within or just deep to the superficial layer of the deep cervical fascia and sometimes are encountered running inferior to the border of the mandible, so care should be taken to preserve

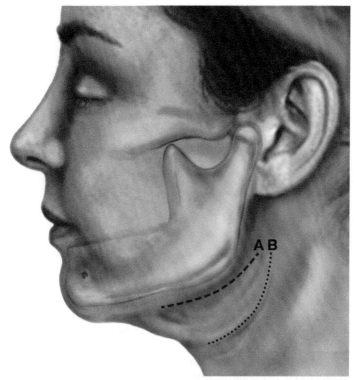

Fig. 2. The incision for the submandibular approach is made 1–2 fingerbreadths below the mandible. Line A shows an incision paralleling the mandible, whereas line B shows an incision made along a skin crease. Placing the incision in a skin crease often improves cosmesis.

it. This can be done by identifying it directly, by only dividing tissue that has been dissected to reveal no nerve, by incising the fascia covering the submandibular gland at its inferior border and elevating it superiorly, or by ligating the facial vein and retracting this superiorly as the marginal mandibular branch is superficial to the facial vein (**Fig. 3**). In many instances, however, the nerve is superior to the area of dissection and is not encountered.

Dissection continues through the deep cervical fascia until the inferior border of the mandible is covered only by periosteum anterior to the premasseteric notch or by the pterogomasseteric sling posterior to the notch. The periosteum or pterogomasseteric sling is divided sharply down to bone and subperiosteal dissection is performed until the fracture site is completely exposed.[3,9,11–13]

Retromandibular Approach

The retromandibular approach provides direct access to the entire posterior ramus and condylar neck and the incision is located proximal to these sites. Potential negatives of this approach include injury to branches of the facial nerve, a visible scar, and potential for a salivary fistula.

There are 2 different retromandibular approaches and the skin incision is marked differently for each one. If a retroparotid approach is desired, then the skin is marked 2 cm posterior to the posterior border of the ramus of the mandible. After incision, the parotid gland is separated from the sternocleidomastoid muscle and then can be

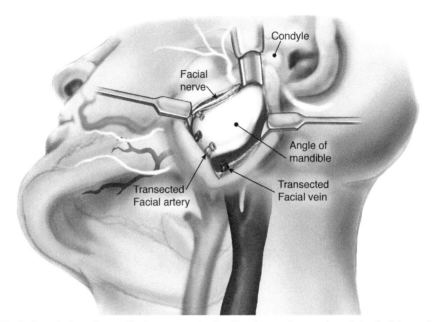

Fig. 3. Seen is the submandibular approach after ligation and retraction of the facial vessels. The pterygomasseteric sling has been elevated off to expose the mandible.

retracted superiorly. The retroparotid approach theoretically has an advantage of protecting the branches of the facial nerve within the parotid gland but negates the advantage of being closer to the ramus and subcondylar regions of the mandible. If a transparotid approach is desired, then the incision is made immediately posterior to the ramus approximately 0.5 cm inferior to the lobule and continues inferiorly for approximately 3 cm to the angle of the mandible. The scant platysma muscle and parotid capsule are then sharply incised. Blunt dissection in an anteromedial direction commences toward the posterior border of the mandible, with all spreads made parallel to the course of the facial nerve branches. Frequently the cervical, marginal mandibular, or buccal branches of the facial nerve are encountered and, if necessary for exposure of the fracture, these branches can be dissected free of tissue for a couple of centimeters and then gently retracted. The pterygomasseteric sling at the posterior border of the mandible is exposed and is incised sharply down to the bone. Subperiosteal dissection with stripping the masseter muscle off of the ramus is then performed to expose the fracture site. Surgeons should always be mindful of the retromandibular vein that runs vertically across the dissection site.[3,9,11]

Intraoral Approach

The traditional intraoral approach often provides poor visualization of the posterior border of the ramus and subcondylar region and it can be difficult to apply fixation plates and screws. Many types of retractors, including lighted retractors, and trocar systems have been developed to help aid in the traditional intraoral approach. Some investigators have also advocated fixating subcondylar fractures with a lag screw, which is easier to apply than plates and screws through the exposure provided by the intraoral approach.[14] The main advantages of the intraoral route are that there are no external incisions or visible scars and that the branches of the facial nerve are not placed at risk.

An incision in made in the ipsilateral gingivobuccal sulcus, preserving a cuff of mucosa medially to facilitate closure. This should start around the second molar and extend posteriorly over the external oblique ridge and further extension along the anterior border of the ramus (**Fig. 4**). The periosteum is incised and a mucoperiosteal flap is raised and reflected to expose the anterior and lateral part of the ramus. Subperiosteal dissection up the anterior edge of the ascending ramus strips the buccinator attachments, which allows the muscle to retract upward, minimizing the chance of herniation of the buccal fat pad. The masseter muscle is stripped off of the lateral surface of the ramus as dissection proceeds superiorly, exposing the condylar neck and sigmoid notch.[9,14]

Endoscopic Approach

The endoscopic approach is the authors' preferred method open treatment for condylar fractures (**Fig. 5**). Arch bars are applied and all other mandibular fractures are treated. A vertical incision is made along the anterior border of the ascending ramus of the mandible. Next, subperiosteal dissection is performed widely, including dissection around the posterior edge of the mandible. This improves mobilization of the fractured segment.

Using a preoperative Panorex, the degree of overlap of the proximal segment on the distal mandible is estimated and a sterile silastic block wedge is cut to this vertical dimension. Patients are placed in heavy elastics across the entire occlusal plane except on the ipsilateral molar region, where this block is wedged while the distal segment is distracted inferiorly. At this point, the adequacy of the reduction is judged with a standard 30° endoscope with irrigating sheath. The authors have found the

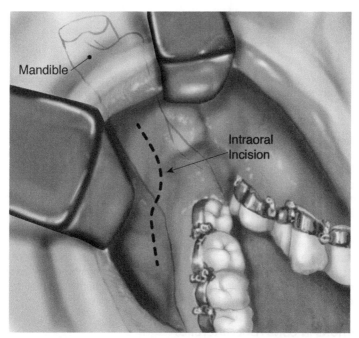

Mandible

Intraoral Incision

Fig. 4. Seen is the incision for the intraoral approach on the right side. This should start lateral to the posterior inferior molars, leaving a cuff of tissue medially to sew to and then extend up onto the ascending ramus of the mandible.

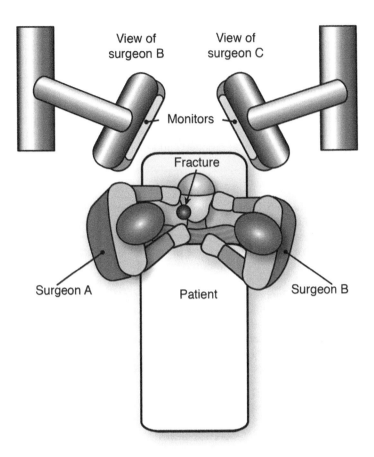

Fig. 5. Schematic view showing 2 surgeons' approach to endoscopic approach. Video towers should be placed behind and adjacent to each surgeon to allow both surgeons to comfortably see.

sheaths used for endobrow lifts invaluable in regards to both irrigation and for tenting up surrounding tissue and improving visualization. Generally, the fracture is well reduced or easily reducible at this juncture. If there is still some overlap present, the silastic block wedge is resized.

Next, the fracture is plated with a 2.0-mm mini–locking screw plate, with 2 screws on either side of the fracture line. Screws are placed through a single transcutaneous stab incision (**Fig. 6**). The screws are placed first on either side of the fracture line with the proximal segment screwed first. The occlusion is verified, and then the outside screws placed. The intraoral incision is closed with a single running layer of 3.0 Vicryl suture. Postoperatively, the patients are mobilized with physiotherapy exercises as soon after fracture fixation as their other injuries allow. Patients are maintained on a no-chew diet for a period of 6 weeks.[6]

COMPLICATIONS IN CONDYLAR FRACTURES

Complications of condylar/subcondylar fractures can be secondary to the original injury as a result of treatment of the fracture or from failure to treat the fracture. These

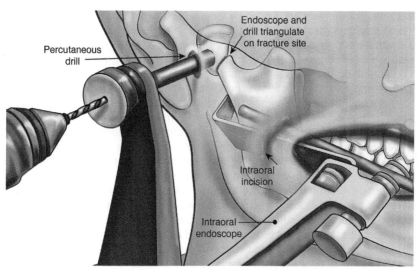

Fig. 6. Endoscopic view showing percutaneous incision with camera in place for direct observation.

complications can be either immediate or long term. Immediate complications include pain, swelling, bleeding, bruising, trismus, nerve damage, loss or damage of teeth or bone, and airway compromise. Airway compromise can be caused from swelling, mandibular displacement, foreign body aspiration, or bleeding, which can be treated with steroids, an oropharyngeal or nasopharyngeal airway, preliminary reduction and immobilization in severely displaced fractures, intubation, or tracheostomy. Also, with the force required to fracture the mandible, it is possible to have other body system injuries that take priority over the mandible fracture, and these should be ruled out with history, physical examination, and other studies, if indicated.[9,15] An immediate complication seen during surgical treatment can be nerve damage. Facial nerve damage is more common in the external approaches used to access the condylar region, such as the preauricular, retromandibular, or submandibular approaches, than in the intraoral approach. Damage to the inferior alveolar nerve can also occur from screw placement into the nerve in the mandibular canal.[15,16]

Long-term complications can result either from a surgical procedure to treat the fracture or from patients not receiving proper treatment. Long-term complications specific to open procedures to reduce and fixate subcondylar fractures include unsightly scars and parotid fistula.[15] The most common long-term complication is infection. Infections involving condyle or subcondylar fractures seem to occur less frequently than other locations of the mandible.[17,18] Some studies have shown that infection rates are higher in open reduction than closed reduction procedures.[18] Risks of developing an infection include delay in treatment, the lack or inappropriate use of antibiotics, teeth in the fracture line, comminution of the fracture, patient noncompliance, inadequate reduction, and concurrent medical problems that inhibit wound healing.[15] Most infections are of minor consequence and can be treated with antibiotics. They do, however, have the potential to develop into more significant sequelae, such as abscess, wound dehiscence, debilitating pain, loose hardware, malunion, nonunion, chronic osteomyelitis, and acquired skeletal deformities.[18] Abscess should be treated with incision and drainage. Hardware might need to be removed and replaced in instances of infection that does not respond to antibiotics or drainage. Osteomyelitis is treated by means of a multistep approach involving incision and drainage, sequestrectomy, frequent irrigations, immobilization, and prolonged antibiotics. In cases of malunion, nonunion, or osteomyelitis nonresponsive to treatments (listed previously) or when bone volume is lost, reconstructive surgery with bone grafting or microvascular surgery may be necessary.[9,15,16]

Another long-term complication is nonunion, which is the lack of an osseous union of 2 or more fractured bone segments after the usual 6-week to 8-week healing period. This can be treated first by conservative management, which consists of prolonged immobilization and optimizing concomitant medical conditions or infections. If this fails, then a second surgical intervention is indicated, which could involve removing soft tissue or teeth that are preventing bone-to-bone contact, removing any infected tissue or bone, and then re-establishing occlusion, reduction, and rigid fixation. Bone grafts might be needed if there is not enough vascularized bone on both sides of the fracture that can be reduced to achieve bone-to-bone contact.[15,17]

Malunion can occur when fractured segments achieve bony union in a less than ideal position because they are not properly reduced or fixated. Because of their anatomic location, malunion of condylar and subcondylar fractures can lead to malocclusion, TMJ arthropathy, decreased lateral excursion, degenerative joint disease, ankylosis, mandibular deviation, and potential growth disturbances.[9,15,16] When malunion is recognized, it should be treated as quickly as possible. Minor malocclusion or malunion can be treated with arch bars, elastic bands, or orthodontic care. More gross abnormalities may require surgery with osteotomies, proper reduction, and re-establishment of proper occlusion.[15]

Other long-term complications include ankylosis, growth disturbance, and condyle resorption. Ankylosis, or fusion of the condyle to the articular fossa, can occur with or without surgery and is more common in the pediatric population. It is generally associated with fractures of the condylar process rather than the subcondylar areas. It can best be avoided by physical therapy regimens initiated as soon as possible and by avoiding long periods of immobilization. Should ankylosis occur, secondary surgical techniques need to be used.[9,16] Because the condyle serves as a growth center for the mandible, a fracture in this area can cause growth disturbance in younger patients, resulting in asymmetry or retrognathia.[9] Condylar resorption, in which the condyle changes shape and decreases in size, can be caused by excessive dissection and injury of the adjacent blood vessels during surgery; it be minimized by careful surgical technique.[16]

POSTPROCEDURAL CARE

Postoperatively, patients are given pain medication and started on Peridex rinse after each meal for 3 days. The authors often also prescribe a short course of an antiemetic and stool softener, to ameliorate the most common postsurgical issues. If the jaw is wired shut, disposable wire cutters are sent home with patients, in case of emesis. A liquid or no-chew diet is also implemented for up to 6 weeks. It is important to council patients and families in regards to typical weight loss associated with closed reduction and the necessity to supplement routine dietary intake. Risks of postoperative smoking and poor wound healing are also reviewed.

REHABILITATION AND RECOVERY

Patients are routinely maintained on a no-chew diet for 6 weeks. If elastic bands are used in closed reduction, then immediate mobilization is encouraged, with slowly increasing jaw mobility and opening. Elastic bands are continued for 3 weeks and with a further 3 weeks of arch bars maintenance before their removal. If instead, wires are used, these are kept in place 2 to 3 weeks and then replaced with elastics and again mobilization is highly encouraged, following the same time course. If there are concerns of continued limited joint mobility, then physiotherapy may be prescribed.

OUTCOMES AND CLINICAL RESULTS IN THE LITERATURE

Debate continues regarding optimal treatment of condylar fractures. Regardless of approach, early mobilization is key to long-term prognosis.[19] Pediatric cases are best treated conservatively. In a review article, Nussbaum and Laskin[20] attempted to more definitively answer whether open or closed is the best approach. Unfortunately, due to significant inconsistencies in measured variables, the investigators were unable to come up with a conclusion. Surgeons are left on their own to interpret the available data and using personal experience to determine the best treatment for our patients.

SUMMARY

There is a role for both open and closed reduction in the treatment of condylar fractures. Using a thoughtful approach with an understanding of the pros and cons of each treatment option, applied individually to each patient fracture, leads to the best long-term outcomes while minimizing the sequelae associated with surgery. Careful unbiased critique of postoperative results with the goal of continually improving techniques and outcomes is, in the end, significantly beneficial to both patients and surgeons.

REFERENCES

1. Ellis E III, Throckmorton G. Treatment of mandibular condylar process fractures: biological considerations. J Oral Maxillofac Surg 2005;63:115–34.
2. Malkin M, Kresberg H, Mandel L. Submandibular approach for open reduction of condylar fractures. Oral Surg Oral Med Oral Pathol 1964;17:152.
3. Landes C, Lipphardt R. Prospective evaluation of a pragmatic treatment rationale: open reduction and internal fixation of displaced and dislocated condyle and condylar head fractures and closed reduction of non-displaced, non-dislocated fractures. Part I: condyle and subcondylar fractures. Int J Oral Maxillofac Surg 2005;34:859–70.
4. Ellis E III, Kellman RM, Vural E. Subcondylar fractures. Facial Plast Surg Clin North Am 2012;20:365–82.
5. Mathes SJ, Hentz VR. Plastic surgery. 2nd edition. Philadelphia: Saunders Elsevier; 2006.
6. Ducic Y. Endoscopic treatment of subcondylar fractures. Laryngoscope 2008; 118:1164–7.
7. Cole P, Kaufman Y, Hollier L. Managing the pediatric facial fracture. Craniomaxillofac Trauma Reconstr 2009;2(2):77–83.
8. He D, Yang C, Chen M, et al. Modified preauricular approach and rigid fixation for intracapsular condyle fracture of the mandible. J Oral Maxillofac Surg 2010;68(7): 1578–84.
9. Montazem AH, Anastassov GA. Management of condylar fractures. Atlas Oral Maxillofac Surg Clin North Am 2009;17:55–69.
10. Ellis E III, Zide MF. Chapter 12 Preauricular approach. Approaches to the facial skeleton. Lippincott Williams & Wilkins; 2006. p. 193–212.

11. Ebenezer V, Ranalingam B. Comparison of approaches for the rigid fixation of subcondylar fractures. J Maxillofac Oral Surg 2011;10(1):38–44.

12. Kanno T, Mitsugi M, Sukegawa S, et al. Submandibular approach through the submandibular gland fascia for treating mandibular fractures without identifying the facial nerve. J Trauma 2010;68(3):641–3.

13. Ellis E III, Zide MF. Chapter 9 Submandibular approach. Approaches to the facial skeleton. 2nd edition. Lippincott Williams & wilkins; 2006. p. 153–68.

14. Patil RS, Gudi SS. Management of subcondylar fracture through intraoral approach with rigid internal fixation. J Maxillofac Oral Surg 2011;10(3):209–15.

15. Zweig BE. Complications of mandibular fractures. Atlas Oral Maxillofac Surg Clin North Am 2009;17:93–101.

16. Choi KY, Yang JD, Chung HY, et al. Current concepts in the mandibular condyle fracture management part I: overview of condylar fracture. Arch Plast Surg 2012; 39:291–300.

17. Stacey DH, Doyle JF, Mount DL, et al. Management of mandible fractures. Plast Reconstr Surg 2006;117(3):48e–60e.

18. Lamphier J, Ziccardi V, Ruvo A, et al. Complications of mandibular fractures in an urban teaching center. J Oral Maxillofac Surg 2003;61:745–9.

19. Zachariades N, Meztis M. Fractures of the mandibular condyle: a review of 466 cases. Literature review, reflections on treatment and proposals. J Craniomaxillofac Surg 2006;34(7):421–32.

20. Nussbaum M, Laskin D. Closed versus open reduction of mandibular condylar fractures in adults: a meta-analysis. J Oral Maxillofac Surg 2008;66:1087–92.

Management of Pediatric Mandible Fractures

Erik M. Wolfswinkel, BS, William M. Weathers, MD,
John O. Wirthlin, DDS, MSD, Laura A. Monson, MD,
Larry H. Hollier Jr, MD*, David Y. Khechoyan, MD

KEYWORDS

- Pediatric mandible fracture • Treatment • Management

KEY POINTS

- Pediatric mandible fractures require a systematic and thorough initial assessment to evaluate the mandibular injury and associated injuries, including cervical spinal injury.
- Management should be performed by a team approach, which includes the plastic surgeon, pediatric dentist, orthodontist, and appropriate consultations to manage associated injuries.
- Most pediatric mandibular fractures can be managed conservatively with a soft diet, analgesics, and movement restrictions.
- The type of treatment modality is often determined by 2 primary considerations: location of fracture and status of dentition.
- Long-term follow-up is required for all pediatric mandible fractures.

BACKGROUND

When determining the optimal treatment strategy for a pediatric mandible fracture, planning must factor in the patient's age, anatomy, stage of dental development, fracture site, and ability to cooperate with the proposed treatment plan. Careful consideration must be given to the possibility of long-term growth disturbances secondary to various fracture locations and types of treatment. As such, the management of a pediatric mandible fracture is substantially different from that of the adult injury.[1–3] This article reviews the current principles of the management of pediatric mandibular fractures.

Financial Disclosures/Commercial Associations: None.
Products/Devices/Drugs: None.
Division of Plastic Surgery, Michael E. Debakey Department of Surgery, Baylor College of Medicine, 6701 Fannin Street, Suite 610, Houston, TX 77030-2399, USA
* Corresponding author.
E-mail address: larryh@bcm.edu

Otolaryngol Clin N Am 46 (2013) 791–806
http://dx.doi.org/10.1016/j.otc.2013.06.007
oto.theclinics.com

EPIDEMIOLOGY

Pediatric mandible fractures account for 32.7% of all facial fractures, followed by nasal bone fractures (30.2%) and midface/zygoma fractures (28.6%).[4] Mandible fractures are rare in the children younger than 5 years.[1–6] The condyle is the most common fracture site in pediatric patients, accounting for 40% to 70% of mandibular fractures. Unilateral condylar fractures are more common than bilateral condylar fractures, with bilateral fractures seen approximately 20% of the time.[7–10] Symphyseal fractures account for approximately 2% to 30% of all mandible fractures. Fractures of the body, angle, and ramus account for the remainder of the fracture locations.[1–5] Symphyseal and parasymphyseal fractures occur more often in children than in adults, which may be partially explained by the presence of developing canine tooth buds resulting in a stress point at the inferior border of the mandible.[9] Following eruption of the canine, bone fills this vulnerable location, making it more durable. On reaching adolescence, fracture-location patterns become similar to those of an adult, with an increase in fractures of the body of the mandible. Multiple fracture sites occur in approximately 40% to 60% of cases and are more frequent in adolescent children.[11–13]

Motor vehicle accidents and falls are responsible for most pediatric mandibular fractures. As children age, a greater proportion of their injuries are associated with sporting accidents. As teenagers (and likewise adults), more fractures are a result of assault.[11,13] Overall, mandible fractures may have a high rate of associated injuries that commonly affect the head, face, and spine. When examining a patient, the physician should carefully evaluate for associated injuries. Studies have shown that greater than 75% of patients with mandibular fracture had additional injuries, including 8% with associated midface fractures.[12,13] Associated midface fractures are more common in adolescent-aged children than in younger children. Whether assessed clinically or with additional imaging, careful evaluation of the cervical spine is a required part of the assessment of a pediatric patient with a traumatic mandible injury.

DEVELOPMENT
Facial Skeleton

Drastic changes in the proportions of the facial skeleton can be seen as the child ages. At birth, the face-to-cranium ratio is 1:8, compared with a ratio of 1:2 in an adult.[14] There is marked growth in the facial skeleton in relation to the rest of the head as the child ages. Vertical growth of the mandible is achieved through bony remodeling along with the development of alveolar process and eruption of the dentition. The posterior borders of the condyle and ramus are particularly active in bone growth with new bone deposition and remodeling, while the anterior surface undergoes bone resorption (**Fig. 1**). There are minimal changes in the body or symphysis of the mandible, with significant growth and remodeling at the ramus and condyle.[15] This process results in a translation forward and downward of the mandible as it grows superiorly and posteriorly, maintaining condylar contact with the glenoid fossa.

The pediatric facial skeleton during early development has many protective features that make it more resilient to withstand traumatic forces. The bones are resistant to fracture because of poor pneumatization, higher elasticity, high ratio of cancellous to cortical bone, and relatively more thick surrounding soft tissue and adipose coverings. The mandible and maxilla also benefit from lying in a relatively more protected position, with additional stability provided by the unerupted dentition. These factors decrease the likelihood of fractures of the mandible and explain why greenstick and condylar fractures are more common in children than in adults.[16]

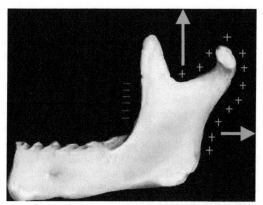

Fig. 1. The posterior borders of the condyle and ramus are particularly active in bone growth and remodeling, while the anterior surface is more susceptible to bone resorption.

As the child develops from an infant to an adolescent, the anatomic relationships of key structures change. The inferior alveolar nerve (IAN) travels adjacent to the lingual cortical surface close to the inferior border of the mandible in younger children. As a child ages and the mandible grows, the nerve progressively becomes more superior in location. This anatomic finding is an important consideration in avoiding injury when placing plate-and-screw fixation.

Dentition

Teeth begin to appear in a child at around 6 months of age. Deciduous teeth gradually erupt until a full complement of 20 primary teeth is seen, at around age 2 years. The primary teeth are relatively stable until age 6, when exfoliation begins to occur and the roots are resorbed. Root resorption causes the crowns of deciduous dentition to loosen and eventually fall out. At around the same time, permanent dentition eruption begins with the initial eruption of central incisors and first molars. Eruption of secondary (permanent) dentition continues through age 12. Children older than 12 years generally have a healthy complement of permanent teeth. The wisdom teeth usually erupt around early adulthood.[17]

During this transition from edentulous stage to mixed dentition stage to permanent dentition stage, the ratio of tooth to bone transitions from high to low. The location of unerupted permanent tooth follicles as an important consideration in terms of where to place plate-and-screw fixation during operative repair of pediatric mandible fractures. Care should be taken to not disrupt the tooth buds. In addition, fractures can occur through the developing tooth crypts, owing to the unerupted teeth having only a very thin cortex overlying this area. If a crypt is fractured or disrupted, devitalization and maldevelopment of the permanent teeth may occur.

PRESENTATION AND WORKUP
Initial Assessment

Initial evaluation of an injured child in whom a facial fracture is suspected begins with a systematic approach and close adherence to Advance Trauma Life Support principles. The primary and secondary trauma surveys should be performed routinely on all patients. A systematic and detailed physical examination is performed to avoid missing any associated injuries.

Based on the mechanism and force of trauma, a child with a traumatic mandibular injury is at risk for associated airway compromise, cervical spinal injury, and neurologic injury. Causes of airway obstruction include direct trauma, swelling, hematoma, or foreign bodies (including aspirated teeth and bone fragments). Often airway obstruction can be managed with patient repositioning, but one needs to remain aware of cervical spine precautions. Suctioning or a finger-sweep technique to remove blood and debris within the oropharynx may also be necessary. Manual anterior traction of the mandibular symphysis or placement of a traction stitch on the tongue may alleviate airway obstruction, particularly in cases where the mandible is displaced posteriorly. Orotracheal intubation or placement of an emergent surgical airway may need to be performed. A spinal injury should be assumed until excluded clinically and/or radiographically. Most patients with facial trauma will undergo computed tomography (CT) scanning to evaluate the facial skeletal injury. Additional CT imaging of cervical spine or head and a modified Glasgow Coma Scale assessment for infants and children to assess neurologic status may be required, depending on mechanism of injury.[18]

Once the patient is stable and a trauma evaluation is complete, a thorough history should be obtained. The patient's allergies, medications, medical and surgical history, timing of last meal, and events surrounding the accident should be obtained. Information regarding the mechanism of injury may help guide the examiner as to the extent of injury. Furthermore, evidence of abuse should be suspected if the narrative of the caregiver's account of the injury does not match the extent and pattern of the injuries.

Physical Examination

Once the trauma evaluation is completed and an open airway is secured, a more focused examination of the injury can be undertaken. A thorough examination of the head and neck should be performed, evaluating the skin, soft tissue, neurovascular structures, and bone. One should begin with an examination of the face and make note of any gross visual asymmetry. Ecchymosis and soft-tissue swelling may be indicators of underlying fracture locations. Lacerations may also provide clues to fracture locations. A chin laceration often indicates a forward fall with a midline force distributed superiorly, which may cause injury to the condyles; this may result in a crush-type injury or displacement of the condyle.

The examiner should then carefully assess the patient for neurologic deficits. Examination of the cranial nerves should be attempted. Particular attention should be given to paresthesias in the forehead, cheek, and lower lip as well as any deficits in facial nerve function. A fracture of the body of the mandible may injure the ipsilateral IAN, resulting in numbness of the chin and teeth. Injuries to the lingual and long buccal nerve have been reported in displaced fractures. Lingual and long buccal nerve injuries result in sensory deficits of the anterior tongue and lip and cheek mucosa, respectively. Nerve injuries that are not carefully documented during the preoperative examination may be later attributed to an iatrogenic complication.

The patient should be asked about how his or her bite feels and about pain, particularly with mandible excursions on mouth opening. Patients are capable of subjectively assessing minute changes in their occlusion and intercuspation. Examining the patient during mouth opening and closure can be quite revealing as to the presence of a fracture and its location. The patient's jaw may deviate or have limited mobility, with decreased maximal incisor opening. Translational movement of the condyle should also be tested by evaluating lateral excursive movements of the mandible. In addition, drooling and trismus may be seen in association with mandible fractures. Trismus is often the result of significant muscle spasm and pain seen after fracture.

Palpation of facial skeleton may reveal step-offs or structural instability. The entire mandible should be palpated intraorally and extraorally. The authors recommend bimanual examination of the mandible, as deviations in symmetry can expose underlying injuries. The insertion of the medial pterygoid muscle on the medial mandibular surface, and the insertion of the temporalis muscle on the coronoid process, should also be assessed for tenderness and mobility. Palpation of the temporomandibular joints while the patient opens and closes the mouth allows for assessment of condyle symmetry, condylar head rotation, and translation of the condyle down the articular eminence. In addition, palpation of the external auditory canal during jaw movement may disclose a displaced condylar head or crepitation. Further examination of the ear may provide evidence for condylar fracture, as these fractures can cause bleeding or ecchymosis of the anterior wall of the external auditory canal.

Examination of the oral cavity is essential, and the patient should be checked for loose teeth, bone fragments, and foreign bodies. The intraoral examination includes evaluation of the entire mouth including teeth, floor of the mouth, tongue, buccal mucosa, vestibular mucosa, and the hard and soft palate. Depending on the patient's age, loose permanent teeth may suggest a fracture along the tooth orientation.

Intraoral examination may be revealing if one is aware of the child's prefracture occlusion status. Evaluation of the occlusion in a pediatric patient can be difficult, especially in a child with mixed dentition. Attention to wear facets, preinjury dental records, and parental input can be helpful in predicting the preinjury occlusion. Minor displacement of the mandible can lead to significant changes in occlusion. Evidence of an anterior open bite indicates bilateral condylar fractures. A unilateral condylar fracture will result in a contralateral posterior open bite. Intraoral examination may also reveal lacerations or hematomas. Antibiotic therapy with appropriate coverage for oral and cutaneous pathogens should be administered if intraoral or through-and-through cutaneous lacerations are present. Any mandible fracture through a tooth-bearing region is considered an "open" fracture, and requires prophylactic antibiotic therapy.

Assessment of dental injuries is also important. Children with permanent dentition injuries require rapid treatment. If teeth are believed to be missing and unaccounted for, a chest radiograph should be obtained as a precautionary measure to evaluate for aspiration. If an intraoral laceration overlying an unerupted tooth occurs, the laceration should be copiously irrigated, and an absorbable suture should be used to reapproximate the mucosa. Every effort should be made to leave the unerupted permanent teeth unscathed.

Imaging

When high clinical suspicion of a mandible fracture is present, further confirmation and characterization of the fracture type, location, and pattern should be performed with radiographic imaging. There are multiple modalities that can be used appropriately in varying situations. These modalities include plain radiographs, panoramic radiograph (orthopantomogram), and CT. Panorex was historically considered to be the study of choice, although this modality has several obvious limitations. A patient needs to be sufficiently cooperative and motionless for Panorex imaging.[11–13,19] Extraneous movements and inaccurate patient position may lead to movement artifact that may conceal a fracture and prevent an accurate diagnosis. Another issue is that a Panorex cannot always be taken with a patient in a supine position. A supine Panorex requires special equipment. If this equipment is unavailable and the patient has spinal precautions, another imaging modality should be used. Often in these cases, a series of plain radiographs are taken. Plain radiographs can provide similar timely information in the acute trauma setting. A mandible series may be obtained, which includes a posteroanterior radiograph, a Townes view, bilateral obliques, lateral view, and often a submentovertex view.[20] In all cases, it is important to obtain multiple views from which a fracture can be visualized in at least 2 planes. Fractures may not be visible in 1 dimension alone. This principle also applies to CT, as axial, sagittal, and coronal cuts allow for more precise and accurate diagnosis. Three-dimensional reconstruction of CT data is also invaluable in evaluating the pattern of injury, and is especially useful in evaluating condylar injuries (**Fig. 2**).[21] Overall CT imaging is the most versatile and clinically useful modality for imaging traumatic mandible injuries, allowing for accurate diagnosis and detailed, targeted treatment planning.

Consults

Based on the presence of associated injuries after completion of detailed physical and imaging assessment, the examiner should involve consulting specialties such as Neurosurgery, Ophthalmology, and Dentistry in a timely fashion. Based on the authors' experience, the care of a child with a traumatic facial injury is best directed by a dedicated trauma team. Presence of such a system ensures appropriate and thorough workup, as well as recruitment of ancillary services such as Social Work and Child Life specialists to assist in the care of the injured child.

Initial Management

When caring for these injuries, operative and nonoperative management as well as inpatient or outpatient management should be determined. Some patients may benefit from a 24-hour overnight observation to assess pain management and oral intake. Others can be managed strictly as outpatients until further intervention is required. These patients are managed conservatively with a soft diet and appropriate analgesics to maintain adequate nutrition and comfort. An oral mouthwash is also provided. If surgical intervention is necessary, it should be completed within the first 7 days. Given the rapid healing potential of children, a longer wait time may make obtaining surgical reduction more difficult, owing to callus formation at the fracture site.

TREATMENT
General Treatment Considerations

Treatment of pediatric mandible fractures during the deciduous and mixed dentitions has remained a topic of debate. Depending on the type and pattern of injury, the

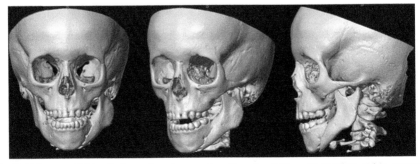

Fig. 2. When available, 3-dimensional reconstruction should be obtained to aid in accurate assessment of the mandible (symphysis, condyles) and associated injuries that are difficult to visualize with other imaging techniques.

treating surgeon may elect a conservative approach with soft diet and observation versus an operative approach. An operative approach, in turn, may involve a spectrum of techniques, such as closed reduction with maxillomandibular fixation (MMF), splinting techniques, or formal open reduction and internal fixation (ORIF).

In all cases, the overriding goal of treatment is restoration of function and preinjury occlusion and reestablishment of facial symmetry, while minimizing disruption of normal mandible growth and development. The type of treatment appropriate to achieve these goals depends on several factors including the location of fracture, displacement of fracture fragments, presence of malocclusion, and stage of dental development.[9,14,22,23]

In general, most nondisplaced pediatric mandible fractures may be managed conservatively with close observation, soft diet, analgesics, and activity precautions.[16] Certain cases may require a short period of MMF for 7 to 14 days to reduce pain and correct minor malocclusions. Malocclusion or significant displacement of fracture fragments requires a more involved approach. The type of treatment modality in these cases is further determined by 2 primary considerations: location of fracture and status of dentition.

As a general guideline, intracapsular condylar fractures and subcondylar fractures without significant malocclusion may be successfully managed with a soft diet and initiation of early range of motion. Occasionally, a brief period (no greater than 7–10 days) of temporary MMF may be appropriate to stabilize the fracture fragments, optimize patient comfort, and allow for bony healing. The concern for postinjury ankylosis dictates the short duration of MMF. Displaced fractures in other locations of the mandible may be managed effectively with a 2.0-mm miniplate placed at the lower mandible border with monocortical screw fixation or acrylic lingual splinting. More detailed management descriptions based on the stage of dental development and fracture location are described here.

Management Considerations Based on Stage of Dental Development

The developmental growth of a child must be considered when managing a pediatric mandible fracture. Treatment of a pediatric mandibular fracture should be performed in an appropriate manner based on the age and available dentition. One of the largest differences in treating a child's maxillofacial traumatic injury is the variable dentition status.

Before age 2 years, children can be considered edentulous because the erupted teeth rarely provide adequate support for fixation. An acrylic splint may be useful in these cases to help immobilize the fracture with the addition of circummandibular wires. The splint may be fixated through either the piriform aperture or a paramedian palatal drill hole to immobilize the jaw.[9,24] Following eruption of the deciduous teeth (age 2–5 years), the teeth may be used for fixation. The conical shape of these teeth is amenable to interdental wiring. Risdon cables or mini-arch bars may be used to treat nondisplaced fractures. During mixed dentition (age 6–12 years), the teeth should be evaluated for stability and strength. Primary tooth roots are being resorbed during this stage, which may lead to presence of loose teeth that are not amenable to MMF use. Combinations of the MMF techniques are used to immobilize the jaw for short durations during this mixed-dentition stage. Primary molars and incisors may serve as anchors for fixation during this time frame. After around age 9, children generally are able to tolerate arch-bar placement, because of the establishment of a majority of their permanent dentition. These children's mandibular injuries are treated with standard MMF with ORIF techniques, as required, similar to those used in adult patients.

Management Considerations Based on Fracture Location

Condylar fractures

In the pediatric patient population, the condyle is the most common site of fracture.[25] These fractures rarely require operative management. Children with condylar fractures generally have adequate range of motion and occlusion. Certain cases may require a short period of MMF for 7 to 14 days to reduce pain and correct minor malocclusions. Surgery should be reserved for those with severely displaced fractures, substantial malocclusion, and cases with dislocation obstructing or limiting mandibular range of movement. In these few indications, a sumandibular or preauricular approach to surgery should be performed, depending on the fracture height within the condyle.[26]

Condylar fractures are classified as intracapsular fractures, high condylar neck fractures, and subcondylar fractures. Intracapsular fractures and high condylar fractures are differentiated by involvement of the articular surface. Intracapsular fractures can result from chin impact that disperses force on the condyles, causing crush-type injuries to the articular disk. High condylar fractures have no articular involvement but are located superior to the sigmoid notch. The force of impact that results in high condylar fractures may also medially dislocate the condyle. High neck fractures demonstrate good regenerative potential and union with conservative management alone. Subcondylar fractures are more caudally located and are the most common type of pediatric mandible fracture; they are generally greenstick fractures and do not require open surgical intervention.

Once the surrounding edema has subsided, emphasis on aggressive physical therapy with early range of motion at the temporomandibular joint (TMJ) is the mainstay of treatment. In younger children, range-of-motion exercises can be accomplished with a large lollipop. In older children, the use of stacked popsicle sticks can be used with a steady increase in number of sticks to increase the incisor opening. This action is taken to prevent TMJ ankylosis and dysfunction. If ankylosis is allowed to occur, it is one of the most difficult complications to remedy. Patients at greater risk for post-traumatic ankylosis of the condyle are children younger than 3 years and those with a prolonged period (usually greater than 3 weeks) of maxillomandibular immobilization.

A condylar fracture may cause concern for disruption of normal mandibular growth. It is not uncommon to see restricted growth on the injured side that results in ipsilateral chin deviation and facial asymmetry.[1–3,5] This condition is more likely to be seen in cases of comminuted intracapsular fracture.[27] This disruption of normal mandibular growth can lead to a malocclusion that did not exist immediately following the traumatic injury or the operative treatment. The abnormal growth is often a result of residual poor mandibular function caused by the fracture. Once this poor growth is noted, the patient should be referred to an orthodontist.

In all cases of condylar fractures, long-term follow-up is important. An orthodontist consult can prove invaluable as an adjunct for treatment, and preoperative planning and preparation.

Symphysis, parasymphysis, and body fractures

Management of fractures in the body of the mandible ranges from conservative management to ORIF, depending on the extent of the injury and amount of displacement of the fracture. Nondisplaced and greenstick fractures are managed conservatively. Manual closed reduction of displaced factures may be achieved with the patient under anesthesia followed by immobilization in MMF. ORIF is frequently required for fractures of the symphysis, body, and angle.

Emphasis on occlusion status is important in these fractures, as several deforming muscle forces may differentially act on this portion of the mandible. Occlusion may initially appear adequate, but these injuries are prone to subsequent displacement owing to the submental muscular pull and masticatory stresses. Therefore, close follow-up with such patients is essential for their care, and any new findings should be fully investigated with reexamination and imaging.

Angle and ramus fractures

Greenstick fractures are common at the angle and can be managed conservatively. Immobilization of the fracture at the angle is slightly more difficult, as it is not amenable to splints. However, if the angle is not significantly displaced, closed reduction with placement of the patient in MMF is typically sufficient to treat most fractures. ORIF is required only in highly comminuted fractures or when an acceptable reduction cannot be achieved with less invasive methods. When plating the angle, the addition of an extraoral incision may be beneficial to achieve appropriate exposure of fracture and to allow for easier instrumentation.[28,29]

Ramus fractures may prove to be more difficult to plate relative to other fractures of the mandible. An external approach or a combined intraoral and extraoral approach may be required. Closed reduction with placement of the patient in MMF or arch bars with elastics may occasionally be sufficient to care for these patients.

Dentoalveolar fractures

Dentoalveolar fractures are common, although the true incidence is unknown because most of these injuries are unreported and treated in an office setting. The maxillary incisors are most commonly injured in the pediatric patient population.[30]

Highly mobile permanent teeth located in the line of the fracture may need to be removed. Avulsed or luxated permanent teeth are considered dental emergencies, as timely treatment is required. The injured tooth needs to be reimplanted within a 1- to 2-hour window from the time of the injury. Replacement of a primary tooth is unnecessary. If a permanent tooth is not avulsed but slightly mobile, soft diet and immobilization with semirigid orthodontic wire can help fixate the teeth for 10 days until healing occurs. Splinting of the mobile deciduous or permanent teeth can also benefit the healing process and salvage the mobile tooth. Intruded primary teeth should be left alone. These teeth will eventually reerupt. Some dentoalveolar injuries can result in malformation of the tooth. Follow-up with a pediatric dentist experienced in treating dental trauma is recommended.

Fractures involving the alveolar aspect of the mandible may be treated with open or closed reduction in similar fashion to those in other regions of the mandible. Immobilization and restoration of occlusion with the use of splints or arch bars is vital to reestablish alveolar-arch continuity. Immobilization is limited to 2 weeks in younger children and up to 4 weeks in adolescents. These patients should undergo long-term follow-up to determine if there has been any disruption of permanent dentition development.

Resorbable versus nonresorbable fixation systems

Use of resorbable fixation systems has become routine in several types of craniofacial reconstruction surgery. These materials provide temporary rigid fixation for bone healing to occur and degrade over time as the reconstructed bone regains strength. These characteristics prove particularly ideal for the pediatric population, in which bone growth and turnover creates potential problems for nonresorbable, permanent plates.

The ideal biodegradable plate is mechanically strong and undergoes resorption within a predictable time frame. Variable chemical compositions of these plates attempt to balance an expedient degradation process while minimizing local foreign-body inflammatory reactions. Advantages of currently available resorbable polylactic and polyglycolic acid plates and screws are their radiolucency and elimination of the need to return for hardware removal. Typically their strength holds for 4 to 6 weeks while the complete degradation process may take 1 to 2 years. However, the application of resorbable plates in pediatric facial fracture treatment, particularly pediatric mandible fractures, is not currently widespread. Data from future studies would be required to examine their utility in treating this patient group. Titanium miniplates are still widely used despite the possible benefits of resorbable plates. Titanium plates demonstrate good long-term biocompatibility, have favorable physical properties, can be easily manipulated intraoperatively to treat the fracture, and have the benefit of several decades of predictable use in facial fracture fixation.[31,32]

Some investigators have advocated for removal of nonresorbable plates following a 3- to 4-month healing period. Others argue that performing an additional surgery may actually cause more harm and disrupt the future development of the mandible. No clear answers are available to settle the debate of whether routine hardware removal is necessary. The effects on growth inhibition are difficult to quantify. The need for hardware removal is primarily dependent on an individual surgeon's preference.

OPERATIVE TREATMENT
Patient Positioning

Procedural treatment of pediatric mandible fractures is best performed in an operating room with appropriate lighting and equipment, and usually under general anesthesia. For young children, even more simple interventions such as splint application or wiring may require some form of sedation.

The child is placed supine on the operating room table with the neck in slight extension and the head resting in a horseshoe headrest in a sniffing position. A nasotracheal tube secured with suture to the membranous portion of nasal septum and sutured over a sponge at the hairline is preferred. This positioning allows for unimpeded access to the oral cavity and more accurate evaluation of occlusion, and facilitates placement of MMF. The oral cavity and teeth are thoroughly cleansed with chlorhexidine gluconate oral rinse, and a moistened throat pack is placed. The surgical field is then sterilely prepared widely to include face, head, and neck, to account for intraoperative manipulation and repositioning of the head.

Placement of Maxillomandibular Fixation

Many stabilization techniques are available to achieve MMF. Unlike in adults who can usually tolerate placement of MMF in an emergency room setting, pediatric patients require anesthesia and sedation.

MMF in a pediatric patient may be more challenging based on the stage of dental development. Deciduous teeth or only partially erupted permanent teeth may not have the proper shape to allow for circumdental wire retention. Fewer teeth and partially loose or exfoliating deciduous teeth during the mixed-dentition phase present additional challenges. In general, in a child with stable primary dentition and in a child in mixed dentition with at least 2 or 3 stable teeth in each arch quadrant, arch-bar application and placement of MMF is feasible.

The surgeon's preference typically determines the type of MMF that is placed. Particular MMF techniques include rapid MMF screws, acrylic splints, circummandibular wires, transnasal wires, Risdon cables, and a combination of resorbable screw with suture. Rapid MMF screws are used by some centers; however, iatrogenic injury to the unerupted tooth follicles is a key concern with this technique.

Acrylic splints are an acceptable form of MMF for edentulous children. Although they provide stability to the mandible, there are several disadvantages to this technique. In a younger, uncooperative child, splints may require multiple rounds of anesthesia for acquisition of impressions and for placement and removal of the splint. Another option for mandible immobilization is a single-arch mandible splint secured with circum-mandibular wires (**Fig. 3**). This technique decreases patient discomfort, as it allows the patient to open the mouth. With this technique the jaw swings freely while maintaining stabilization[23]; however, specific expertise and appropriate materials are required to fabricate these splints in a timely manner in the operating room.

Placement of circum-mandibular wires makes use of a small, 3-mm submental stab incision through which a sharp awl is passed intraorally, tightly hugging the lingual cortex of mandible. A 26-gauge or 24-gauge wire is placed through the opening in the tip of the awl, and the awl is partially withdrawn and passed over the anterior or buccal mandible cortex into the gingivobuccal sulcus. This action creates a wire loop around the mandible symphysis and parasymphysis. Care should be exercised in younger children in passing the awl, as portions of the symphysis may be cartilaginous, which may lead to inadvertent passing of the awl through, instead of around the cartilage. The circum-mandibular wire then may be attached to a transnasal wire placed either at the piriform rim or through a paramedian palatal drill hole to immobilize the mandible to the maxilla.[24]

Risdon cables are fabricated from long 24-gauge circumdental stainless-steel wires that are twisted into an arch-bar substitute. Its benefits are that it is low profile, malleable, and can be formed to fit the short bulbous teeth of younger children. The cable is secured to each tooth with 26-gauge circumdental wires similarly to how an arch bar would be fixed. This technique can be manipulated to immobilize several fracture types.[23]

A combination of resorbable screw and suture has been used in multiple locations to immobilize the mandible. Using screws placed in each zygoma following the elevation of a small mucoperiosteal flap has been described. A 0 or 2-0 monofilament suture is passed through a hole in the screw head and then passed around the mandible. The suture is then pulled tight and tied, which creates a sling to fixate the mandible. More medial placement of the screw in the maxilla has also been described (**Fig. 4**). Care should be taken not to disrupt unerupted tooth buds if operating in this location. The screw and suture technique allows for easy release of fixation, as one only needs to cut and remove the suture. This technique may not be appropriate for older children, as the muscle forces exerted on the mandible may overcome the strength of the suture.

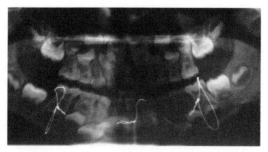

Fig. 3. Mandible immobilization with a single-arch mandible splint secured with circum-mandibular wires.

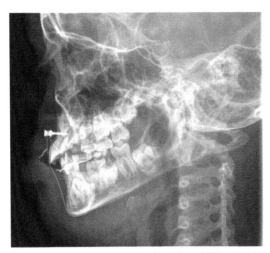

Fig. 4. Mandible immobilization with a screw-and-stitch technique and medial placement of the screw.

Open Reduction and Internal Fixation

Indications for formal ORIF for pediatric mandible trauma are rare, and include complex, multipart fractures of the tooth-bearing regions of mandible, fracture-dislocations of condyle with dislocation into middle cranial fossa, and bilateral condylar fractures with an anterior open bite malocclusion that cannot be reduced and immobilized with MMF alone. An intraoral approach is the preferred access to most fractures. A combined intraoral and extraoral, transfacial approach may be required in some patients. Preauricular incisions extending into the hairline may be needed for displaced condylar injuries.

In general, an inferior-border 2.0-mm plate with monocortical screws is the preferred method of fixation. Plating of the mandibular symphysis can generally be safely performed in mixed-dentition phase after eruption of the central incisors. Plating at the parasymphysis may be safely performed after around age 9, following eruption of the permanent mandibular canines. With monocortical screw fixation using 4-mm screws, plating in the symphysis, parasymphysis, and body regions of the mandible may still be safely accomplished even in patients in whom eruption of the incisors or canines has not fully occurred. A single, lower-border plate is typically sufficient, especially when combined with an arch bar serving as an additional point of fixation. Care should be exercised to place the plate directly on the most inferior aspect of the anterior mandibular border to avoid injury to unerupted tooth follicles and the low-lying IAN in a pediatric patient. In an older pediatric patient, these concerns lessen.[14,23]

After injection of the gingivobuccal sulcus incision with epinephrine-containing local anesthetic, an incision is made to maintain a submucosal and a muscle cuff on the part of the incision close to attached gingiva for ease of approximation during closure. The mandible is exposed in a subperiosteal plane widely to allow for ease of instrumentation.

Care is taken to prevent injury to the mental nerve as it emerges from the foramen; occasionally, to allow for ease of retraction, the periosteal sheath surrounding the nerve may need to be carefully incised and the nerve dissected free of surrounding tissue.

Once the fracture is exposed, irrigation is applied. Any fibrin clot or fracture hematoma within the fracture site is thoroughly debrided to allow for segment mobilization and manipulation. Before reduction and fixation when multiple fractures are present, all fractures are exposed widely with subperiosteal dissection.

Following fracture exposure, the patient is placed into MMF with careful inspection of wear facets on the occluding teeth and seating of mandible condyles within the glenoid fossae. The fracture fragments are reduced and plated only after the preinjury occlusion is established. Bigonial pressure may need to be applied if significant splaying of mandible angles is present.

Reduction of the fractured segments may be challenging in a pediatric patient, as interference from tooth follicles may be present. Occasionally the fracture may have a greenstick component on the opposite (lingual) cortex, which may interfere with adequate reduction. Because of significant anticipated postoperative bony remodeling and rapid healing in children, if the preinjury occlusion is reestablished a small osseous gap at the fracture site may be tolerated and is usually not of any consequence.

Miniplate fixation should be used after establishing preinjury occlusion in MMF. The use of monocortical screws is important in situations when the dentition is in jeopardy. When placing the drill holes, care should be taken to avoid further disruption of the tooth buds.[33] The lateral bony cortex surrounding the tooth bud is approximately 1 mm in thickness, and screws can easily injure the underlying developing tooth follicles. If necessary, a longer plate can be used to avoid drill holes in areas of dentition. For all types of fractures regardless of location, typically at least 2 screws should be placed on either side of the fracture for stable fixation.

After ORIF is applied, the MMF is released. Mandible excursions, seating of the bilateral condyles, and occlusion at wear facets is rechecked. If the occlusion is off or if the condyle is not appropriately seated, the fixation is removed and the sequence of steps is repeated. If successful, MMF may be removed leaving only the arch bars in place. The arch bars serve as an additional point of fixation, similar to a tension band on the mandible, and allow for postoperative placement of elastics if malocclusion or open bites are present. A bridle wire ligating the teeth around the fracture line can also serve as a tension band.[8]

POSTOPERATIVE CARE CONSIDERATIONS

Although a child's greater osteogenic and remodeling potential, and rapid healing response allow tolerance of minor malocclusions and small gaps at the fracture site, all attempts should be made to reestablish preinjury occlusion, even if this requires redoing removal of MMF and repeat of ORIF. When occlusion is considered adequate, the mouth should be copiously irrigated. The intraoral incision is closed with a combination of running or interrupted Vicryl suture, with care to evert the mucosa at the incisions. For the symphyseal and parasymphyseal region, the mentalis muscle should be resuspended with a buried muscle suture, to prevent a secondary chin ptosis and a "witch's chin" deformity. The throat pack is removed, and the oropharynx and stomach are suctioned with a nasogastric tube.

The patient is typically extubated at the end of the operation. The patient is admitted to the hospital for postoperative analgesia, intravenous antibiotics for 24 hours, and monitoring of oral intake. If the patient is left in MMF, wire cutters should be left at the bedside, and the nursing personnel and the caregiver should be instructed on how to release the MMF wires to gain access to the patient's airway in case of an emergency. If the patient who is left in MMF vomits after the operation, the patient should be promptly turned on his or her side, and a suction catheter should be passed behind the maxillary tuberosity into the oropharynx.

If patient is left in MMF, once discharged from hospital the patient and/or caregiver should have the wire cutters on hand at all times. Oral intake for the patient who is left in MMF may be accomplished with passage of a straw through the gap between teeth if present, or with a right-angle straw passed behind the maxillary tuberosity. The parents and patients are counseled that some weight loss (5–10 lb [2.27–4.53 kg]) may result during the period of MMF. Calorie-dense foods such as milkshakes or protein shakes are recommended to allow for weight maintenance and adequate nutrition for healing at the fracture site.

After a brief period of MMF (usually 7–14 days) the arch bars and wires may be removed under brief sedation in the operating room, usually without the need for a general anesthetic.

COMPLICATIONS

Complications are uncommon in this patient population in comparison with adults.[14,16,29] Complications seen with mandibular fractures include:

- Infection
- Malunion
- Nonunion
- Malocclusion
- Facial asymmetry
- Mandibular growth disturbances
- Disruption of permanent teeth
- TMJ dysfunction

Because of concerns for these issues, close postoperative short-term and long-term follow-up are recommended. These children often require orthodontics and, at times, additional surgical intervention.[3,9]

Patients who exhibit persistent malocclusion after unilateral or bilateral condylar fractures that have been treated with MMF can often further be treated nonsurgically; however, some type of functional therapy is recommended to address the abnormal occlusal relationship. This functional therapy can be as simple as elastics in conjunction with orthodontic appliances or occlusal splints, or it may require a formal functional appliance. There is a variety of functional appliances, which are placed by orthodontists, each with advantages and disadvantages, although the goals of all such appliances are the same. Functional appliances seek to mechanically reposition the jaw into proper occlusion and promote proper mandibular function. In growing children, over a period of time, a functional appliance can correct a malocclusion caused by a condylar fracture and help correct abnormal mandibular function.

Growth disturbances in the pediatric patient population have been thoroughly studied. Although the injuries typically heal with significant improvement and function, patients and their parents must be cognizant of the possibility of long-term growth restriction. These patients should be referred to an orthodontist as soon as abnormal growth is noted. Abnormal growth results in facial asymmetry and deviation of the chin, and may not become apparent for several years. The cause of the actual growth disturbances remains unclear, as different outcomes occur with similar fractures. It is possible that certain children may have lost growth stimuli or suffer from decreased regional vascularity, resulting in growth restriction. Maintaining appropriate range of motion at the TMJ is important in maintaining proper mandibular growth, as well as avoiding ankylosis and TMJ dysfunction. In all cases, restoring facial symmetry is a very difficult challenge in these patients, and may require additional interventions that may range from fat grafting, to orthodontics, to combined orthodontic-orthognathic surgery approaches.

Traumatic injuries to areas of active bony growth and remodeling are more susceptible to growth disturbances leading to facial asymmetry and malocclusion. Posttraumatic deformities may require eventual orthodontic or combined orthodontic-orthognathic treatment to correct facial asymmetry and malocclusion. As shown in a study by Demianczuk and colleagues,[3] traumatic mandible injuries in children younger than 4 years or older than 12 years rarely require orthognathic surgery to correct any resulting deformity. By contrast, 22% of children aged 4 to 7 years and 17% of children aged 8 to 11 years required combined orthodontic-orthognathic treatment at skeletal maturity to correct posttraumatic facial asymmetry and malocclusion.[3]

SUMMARY

Treatment of a pediatric patient with a traumatic mandible injury requires precise knowledge of mandibular anatomy, understanding of the effects of dentition on management, and technical expertise in applying different technical strategies based on fracture location and pattern. Treatment is aimed primarily at reestablishing preinjury occlusion and function. Restoration of facial symmetry and mandible contour is the other key aim. Most fractures may be managed conservatively or with a minimally invasive approach, with only a few requiring formal, definitive ORIF. Close short-term and long-term postoperative follow-up is critical for early identification of complications or secondary deformities.

REFERENCES

1. Ferreira PC, Amarante JM, Silva PN, et al. Retrospective study of 1251 maxillofacial fractures in children and adolescents. Plast Reconstr Surg 2005;115:1500–8.
2. Davison SP, Clifton MS, Davison MN, et al. Pediatric mandibular fractures: a free hand technique. Arch Facial Plast Surg 2001;3:185–9.
3. Demianczuk AN, Verchere C, Phillips JH. The effect on facial growth of pediatric mandibular fractures. J Craniofac Surg 1999;10:323–8.
4. Imahara SD, Hopper RA, Wang J, et al. Patterns and outcomes of pediatric facial fractures in the United States: a survey of the National Trauma Data Bank. J Am Coll Surg 2008;207(5):710–6.
5. Schweinfurth JM, Koltai PJ. Pediatric mandibular fractures. Facial Plast Surg 1998;14:31–44.
6. Lindahl L, Hollender L. Condylar fractures of the mandible. II. A radiographic study of remodeling processes in the temporomandibular joint. Int J Oral Surg 1977;6:153–65.
7. Hurt TL, Fisher B, Peterson BM, et al. Mandibular fractures in association with chin trauma in pediatric patients. Pediatr Emerg Care 1988;4:121–3.
8. Smartt JM Jr, Low DW, Bartlett SP. The pediatric mandible: II. Management of traumatic injury or fracture. Plast Reconstr Surg 2005;116:28e–41e.
9. Goth S, Sawatari Y, Peleg M. Management of pediatric mandible fractures. J Craniofac Surg 2012;23(1):47–56.
10. Norholt SE, Krishnan V, Sindet-Pedersen S, et al. Pediatric condylar fractures. J Oral Maxillofac Surg 1993;51:1302–10.
11. Rowe NL. Fractures of the jaws in children. J Oral Surg 1969;27(7):497–507.

12. Thoren H, Iizuka T, Hallikainen D. Different patterns of mandibular fractures in children. An analysis of 220 fractures in 157 patients. J Craniomaxillofac Surg 1992;20(7):292–6.

13. Kaban LB, Mulliken JB, Murray JE. Facial fractures in children: an analysis of 122 fractures in 109 patients. Plast Reconstr Surg 1977;59(1):15–20.

14. Cole P, Kaufman Y, Izaddoost S, et al. Principles of pediatric mandibular fracture management. Plast Reconstr Surg 2009;123(3):1022–4.

15. Proffit WR, Fields HW, Sarver DM. Contemporary orthodontics. 4th edition. St Louis (MO): Mosby Inc; 2007.

16. Siy RW, Brown RH, Koshy JC, et al. General management considerations in pediatric facial fractures. J Craniofac Surg 2011;22(4):1190–5.

17. Smartt JM Jr, Low DW, Bartlett SP. The pediatric mandible: I. A primer on growth and development. Plast Reconstr Surg 2005;116:14e–23e.

18. Morray JP, Tyler DC, Jones TK, et al. Coma scale for use in brain-injured children. Crit Care Med 1984;12:1018–20.

19. MacLennan WD. Fractures of the mandible in children under the age of six years. Br J Plast Surg 1956;9:125–8.

20. Ellis E III, Miles BA. Fractures of the mandible: a technical perspective. Plast Reconstr Surg 2007;120(7):76s–89s.

21. Chacon GE, Dawson KH, Myall RW, et al. A comparative study of 2 imaging techniques for the diagnosis of condylar fractures in children. J Oral Maxillofac Surg 2003;61:668–72.

22. Myall RW. Management of mandibular fractures in children. Oral Maxillofac Surg Clin North Am 2009;21(2):197–201.

23. Kushner GM, Tiwana PS. Fractures of the growing mandible. Atlas Oral Maxillofac Surg Clin North Am 2009;17(1):81–91.

24. McNichols CH, Hatef DA, Cole PD, et al. Optimizing pediatric interdental fixation by use of a paramedian palatal fixation site. J Craniofac Surg 2012;23:605–7.

25. MacLennan WD. Consideration of 180 cases of typical fractures of the mandibular condylar process. Br J Plast Surg 1952;5:122–8.

26. Zide MF. Open reduction of mandibular condyle fractures: indications and technique. Clin Plast Surg 1989;16:69–76.

27. Lund K. Mandibular growth and remodeling processes after condylar fracture: a longitudinal roentgenographic-cephalometric study. Acta Odontol Scand Suppl 1974;32(64):64–71.

28. Zimmermann CE, Troulis MJ, Kaban LB. Pediatric facial fractures: recent advances in prevention, diagnosis and management. Int J Oral Maxillofac Surg 2005;34:823–33.

29. Luhr HG. Fractures of the mandible in children. Oper Techn Plast Reconstr Surg 1998;5(4):357–61.

30. Wilson S, Smith GA, Preisch J, et al. Epidemiology of dental trauma treated in an urban pediatric emergency department. Pediatr Emerg Care 1997;13:12–5.

31. Bell RB, Kindsfater CS. The use of biodegradable plates and screws to stabilize facial fractures. J Oral Maxillofac Surg 2006;64:31–9.

32. Bos RR. Treatment of pediatric facial fractures: the case for metallic fixation. J Oral Maxillofac Surg 2005;63:382–4.

33. Landes CA, Day K, Glasl B, et al. Prospective evaluation of closed treatment of nondisplaced and nondislocated mandibular condyle fractures versus open reposition and rigid fixation of displaced and dislocated fractures in children. J Oral Maxillofac Surg 2008;66(6):1184–93.

Dentoalveolar Trauma

Christopher R. Olynik, DMD, FRCD(C), Austin Gray, DDS,
Ghassan G. Sinada, DDS*

KEYWORDS

- Facial reconstruction • Facial trauma • Dental trauma • Craniomaxillofacial
- Dentition

KEY POINTS

- Dentoalveolar trauma is seen by all individuals treating facial trauma.
- Although the long-term follow-up of the dentition may lie beyond the scope of facial trauma surgeons, important steps can be taken to improve dentoalveolar structure prognosis and treatment outcome.
- The intent of this article is to provide an overview of treatment of dental injuries as encountered in the emergency department.
- Timely referral to a general/pediatric dentist or endodontist is appropriate in almost all cases.
- Consultation with an oral and maxillofacial surgeon is also indicated for immediate treatment as well as for a discussion centered on dental implant reconstruction of the area should it be required.

INTRODUCTION

Dentoalveolar injuries are an important and common component of craniomaxillofacial trauma.[1–13] The dentition serves as a vertical buttress of the face and fractures to this area may result in malalignment of facial subunits. Furthermore, the dentition is succedaneous with 3 phases—primary dentition, mixed dentition, and permanent dentition—mandating different treatment protocols. This article is written for nondental providers to diagnose and treat dentoalveolar injuries.

ANATOMY

The primary dentition and permanent dentition are housed within the alveolar bone of the maxilla and mandible (**Fig. 1**). The quantity of alveolar bone is dependent on the presence and health of teeth as forces are transmitted through the surrounding

Department of Otolaryngology, Greater Baltimore Medical Center, Physicians Pavilion West, 6569 North Charles Street, Suite 601, Baltimore, MD 21204, USA
* Corresponding author.
E-mail address: gsinada@me.com

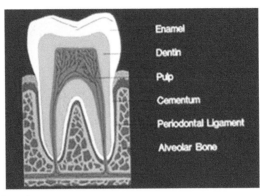

Fig. 1. Basic dental anatomy.

periodontal ligament (PDL). Basal bone comprises the remainder the maxilla and mandible.

Blood supply to mandibular alveolus is mainly from the terminal branches of the internal maxillary artery with contributions from the branches of the facial and lingual arteries. The maxillary alveolus receives its vascular supply from the internal maxillary, ascending pharyngeal, and lingual tonsillar twig arteries. As inferred from the studies by Bell, the redundant nature of the vascular supply allows most dentoalveolar bony injuries to heal well despite mucosal lacerations and extensive comminution. Vascular supply must be considered, however, in incision design when significant trauma is present.

The dentition is innervated by the third division of the trigeminal nerve. The posterior trunk of the mandibular nerve gives rise to the inferior alveolar nerve that enters the mandibular foramen and continues in the inferior alveolar canal. This nerve splits at the mental foramen where a portion exits to innervate the lip and mandibular labial mucosa, and a portion continues on as the incisive branch to innervate the mandibular incisors. The mandibular teeth and their PDLs receive their vascular supply and innervation by way of nutrient canals from this inferior alveolar canal. The lingual, long buccal, and mylohyoid nerves also contribute to innervation of the mandibular dentition and alveolus. The maxillary teeth are innervated by the maxillary nerve by way of the posterior superior alveolar, middle superior alveolar, and anterior superior alveolar nerves. The palatal alveolus receives innervation from the greater and lesser palatine nerves as well as from the terminal branches of the nasopalatine nerve. Accessory and anatomic variations are common.

Teeth are divided into a crown and a root. The crown consists of an outer shell of enamel over dentin that is replete with tubules that connect to the innermost pulp tissues. The pulp tissue contains blood vessels, nerves, and stem cells and may become calcified with trauma or infectious insult. The roots consist of the same basic layers; however, cementum with Sharpey fibers that connect directly to bone replaces the enamel. In addition, there are numerous accessory canals that travel from the root pulp to the PDL to create a complex network of dental vascular supply and innervation. As tooth roots continue to develop, they lengthen and change from an open or immature apex to a closed or mature apex.

The PDL surrounding teeth consist of 9 groups of collagenous fibers that transmit the forces of mastication to the surrounding bone and gingival soft tissue. Radiographically, teeth sit in a socket lined with cortical bone referred to as the lamina dura. The bone on the buccal and lingual aspects of the roots are referred to as the buccal and lingual plates. Normal healthy gingival tissue consists of a band of keratinized tissue near the crowns of teeth and loose alveolar mucosa covering the remainder of the alveolus.

The primary dentition begins erupting between 6 and 12 months of age and results in 20 teeth with spacing that is normal and desirable. The permanent dentition commences with the eruption of the 6-year first molars and continues into the late teenage years and 20s as the third molars complete formation for a total of 32 teeth. The mixed dentition stage represents a transition between the primary dentition and permanent dentition and may result in unstable occlusal schemes. Understanding this basic dental anatomy is important in the diagnosis, treatment options, and prognosis associated with dentoalveolar injuries.

Based on anatomy, dentoalveolar injuries may be divided into several categories. First, injuries to the primary dentition and permanent dentition are treated in a different manner. Second, the extent of tooth structure injured must be evaluated in conjunction with amount of root development. Last, the degree of involvement of the alveolar bone must be considered, with a greater extent requiring principles more akin to fracture treatment.

INJURY TO THE PRIMARY DENTITION

Dental trauma, especially in children, can be a challenging experience for any practitioner from a patient management standpoint. An attempt is made to break this complex issue down into a systematic approach to simplify and improve patient outcomes, written with the intent of being a useful guide to practical treatment in hospital-based emergency settings.

For the sake of this discussion, children are defined as anyone possessing succedaneous teeth or in the primary dentition who is not an adult with retained primary teeth. Complete exfoliation of the primary dentition generally is complete at approximately age 12. As discussed previously, the maturation of a child's permanent dentition and root development greatly affect treatment outcomes. The various functions of primary teeth include

- Space maintenance for permanent tooth eruption
- Alignment and spacing of the permanent dentition
- Occlusion
- Phonetics
- Self-esteem
- Nutritional intake/diet

If the developing permanent teeth are jeopardized by forceful movement of primary teeth in the alveolus, however, preservation of the primary dentition is secondary.

The primary dentition, with 20 teeth in total, are named in the United States starting from the maxillary rightmost posterior secondary primary molar as A around the arch to maxillary left secondary molar as J, with the mandibular left secondary molar commencing with K and continuing through the alphabet to T at the mandibular right secondary molar. In general, eruption (**Fig. 2**) begins at 6 months in anterior mandible and is complete at 30 months with the eruption of the primary secondary molars. A rule of 4 teeth erupting every 7 months can be used to evaluate and assess sequence. A child then progresses until approximately age 5 with minimal changes apparent intraorally until the first permanent molars erupt posterior to the secondary primary molars. The anterior dentition transitions at approximately age 8 to 9 years with completion of exfoliation of the primary dentition at approximately age 12. In general, the entire permanent dentition has erupted by age 18 to 21 years, including the third molars.

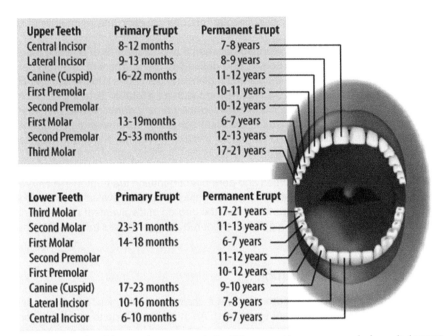

Upper Teeth	Primary Erupt	Permanent Erupt
Central Incisor	8-12 months	7-8 years
Lateral Incisor	9-13 months	8-9 years
Canine (Cuspid)	16-22 months	11-12 years
First Premolar		10-11 years
Second Premolar		10-12 years
First Molar	13-19 months	6-7 years
Second Premolar	25-33 months	12-13 years
Third Molar		17-21 years

Lower Teeth	Primary Erupt	Permanent Erupt
Third Molar		17-21 years
Second Molar	23-31 months	11-13 years
First Molar	14-18 months	6-7 years
Second Premolar		11-12 years
First Premolar		10-12 years
Canine (Cuspid)	17-23 months	9-10 years
Lateral Incisor	10-16 months	7-8 years
Central Incisor	6-10 months	6-7 years

Fig. 2. Primary dentition and permanent dentition eruption sequence (acknowledgment: Partners in dental care).

TOOTH ERUPTION

Of considerable importance, permanent tooth buds/permanent dentition form in alveolus close to the tongue or lingually and erupt generally into the pediatric root structure (laterally) and resorb it slowly until exfoliation occurs or the tooth erupts adjacent to the primary tooth with no exfoliation. This lends to the primary goal of treatment of dentoalveolar trauma in the primary dentition, which is to avoid injury or insult to the developing permanent tooth and to avoid precipitation of significant malocclusion from management of dentoalveolar trauma.

INCIDENCE OF TRAUMATIC INJURIES IN CHILDREN

Children exhibit a bimodal distribution in trauma to the oral cavity, with falls the primary mechanism of injury occurring when a child is beginning to become mobile. According to Andreasen and colleagues, a second peak occurs at age 8 to 10 years with a 2:1 male-to-female ratio as sports become more physical. Child abuse is, unfortunately, another significant cause. In a 2000 review of 879,000 documented US child abuse cases, 19.3% were physical abuse, with 50% of these involving trauma to the head and/or neck. Internationally, approximately 7% of all childhood injuries involve the oral cavity. Concern should arise when the accident and narrative of the accident do not correlate well.

INJURY CLASSIFICATION SCHEMES

Many dentoalveolar trauma classification systems have been developed (**Figs. 3–6**). It is useful to discuss and use them for communication with other health care providers and in documentation of the nature and extent of the injury for medicolegal reasons.

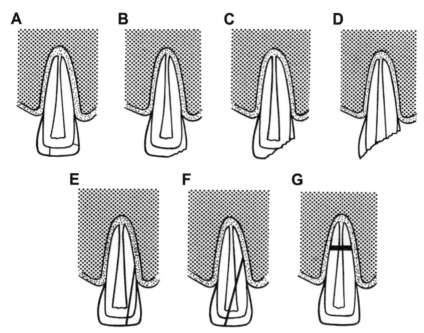

Fig. 3. Infraction (*A*), uncomplicated enamel limited fracture (*B*), uncomplicated crown fracture (*C*), complicated crown fracture (*D*), uncomplicated crown-root fracture (*E*), complicated crown-root fracture (*F*), and root fracture (*G*).

Two of the most common classification schemes are discussed, Ellis/Davey and Andreasen.

Andreasen (Equally Applicable to Primary Dentition and Permanent Dentition)

Dental hard tissue
  Infraction
    Craze/crack in enamel only
    Crown of tooth intact and normal
    Percussion test nontender, normal radiograph
  Uncomplicated enamel limited fracture
    A fracture or chip of enamel only
    Nontender to palpation, nonmobile, enamel loss visible on radiograph
  Uncomplicated crown fracture
    Crown fracture with missing tooth structure, including enamel and dentin but no pulpal or root exposure
  Complicated crown fracture
    Crown fracture through enamel and dentin with exposure of pulp tissues
  Uncomplicated crown-root fracture
    Fracture through enamel, dentin, and cementum without exposure of pulp tissues
  Complicated crown-root tracture
    Fracture through enamel, dentin, and cementum and with pulp tissue exposure
  Root fracture
    Dentin and cementum fractured and pulp tissue exposed to PDL or oral cavity with no fracture of enamel; classified based on coronal third, middle third, or apical third of tooth involved

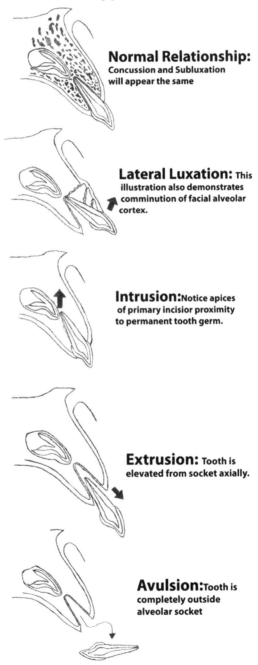

Fig. 4. Injuries to the PDL and alveolar supporting structures.

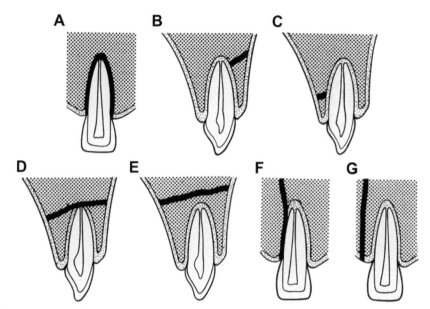

Fig. 5. Patterns of alveolar fracture.

Injuries to PDL/dental supporting structures
  Concussion
  - Injury to PDL producing sensitivity to percussion with no loosening or displacement of the tooth
  Subluxation
  - Tooth loosened in socket but not displaced, sensitive to percussion
  Extrusion
  - Tooth loosened and partially displaced out of socket axially
  - Radiographically widened PDL space at apex of tooth
  - PDL separated from alveolar bone
  Lateral luxation
  - Displacement of tooth other than axially (ie, medially, laterally, anteriorly, or posteriorly)
  - Radiographically, PDL space widened on side of tooth that was displaced away from
  Intrusion
  - Axial displacement of tooth deeper into the alveolus
  - No PDL space evident radiographically
  - Tooth may appear shorter clinically
  - Percussion yields a high-pitched "ting" metallic sound or sound more solid relative to other teeth
  - Can be problematic with primary dentition
  Avulsion
  - Complete disarticulation of tooth from socket

Injuries to supporting bone
  Comminution of both alveolar cortices
    Often with intrusive or lateral luxation

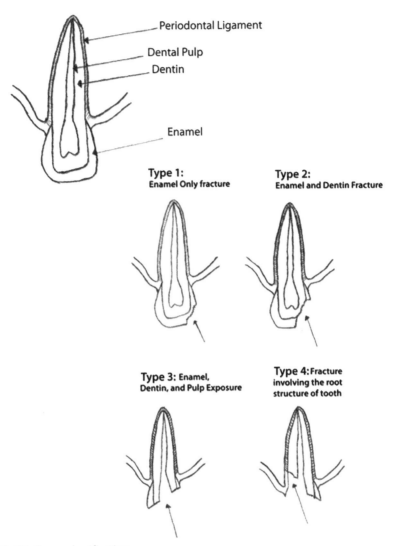

Fig. 6. Ellis/Davey classification.

Fracture of a single cortex
    Buccal or lingual cortex fracture
Fracture of alveolar process en bloc
    Fracture may or may not propagate through socket, may contain 1 or multiple
    teeth but underlying maxilla or mandible grossly stable
Mandible or maxillary fracture

Ellis/Davey

Type 1: fracture limited to enamel
Type 2: fracture of enamel and dentin
Type 3: fracture of enamel, dentin, and pulpal tissue exposure
Type 4: fracture involving the root structure of a tooth

EXAMINATION OF THE TRAUMATIZED CHILD

Pediatric patients' cooperativeness varies greatly as do the extent of injuries that often accompany dentoalveolar injuries. Depending on the mechanism of the injury, a child may have suffered intracranial injuries, be unconscious or intubated, or be a horribly anxious and frightened toddler or a stoic preteen in mixed dentition. Standard advanced trauma life support protocols are followed to assess for life-threatening and acute conditions. Examination and treatment may need to be performed under sedation or general anesthesia.

Best practices dictate instituting a systematic examination record or dentoalveolar trauma record to avoid missing injuries to the oral cavity. No one way or form is superior but the following needs to be addressed in the record. A comprehensive history and physical examination with care to include the following is generally adequate for medicolegal and treatment purposes.

- Description of the incident including cause, location, and time
- Neurologic status, including level of consciousness, presence of headache, nausea, vomiting, and so forth
- Extraoral findings, including other facial trauma
- Intraoral findings
  - Best accomplished with good lighting and suction, examining all soft tissues for ecchymosis, hematomas, and lacerations
  - Care must be taken to identify debris in the oral cavity and account for lost dentition, appliances, or other hardware that evidence seems to indicate might have possibly been dislodged and is not accounted for in its entirety
  - Chest and abdominal imaging should be ordered as indicated

Tooth Vitality Testing

Most investigators argue that tooth vitality testing is not especially accurate or useful in the primary dentition with open root apices or based on verbal response from patients (skewed by age, ability to communicate, and sedation).

Tooth Mobility

Mobility is usually classified based on the Miller system. Simply put, gentle pressure is directed with a cotton tip applicator (1–2 lb pressure), or some other device besides the practitioner's finger, in anterior-posterior, mediolateral, and apical directions. Miller 1+ is perceived gross tooth movement but less than 1 mm, 2+ is perceived movement greater than 1 mm but no vertical or axial movement, and 3+ is 2+ criteria except vertical/axial gross mobility is perceived.

Classification of Dental Injury of Each Tooth Based on Ellis/Davey or Andreasen

Percussion is especially useful when dealing with subacute or poor historians who are unable to indicate if their dentition has been injured. It can be accomplished in an emergency department with a blunt metal object that transmits small amounts of force to teeth efficiently, such as a dental mirror handle. The premise is to compress the PDL space underlying teeth. First, an unaffected control site is tested by gently raising the instrument 5 mm to 8 mm above the tooth and striking it on its occlusal or incisal edge. The force used to percuss teeth should not exceed what is comfortable to perform on a proximal nail fold of an index finger when supported on a rigid object. Time should be taken to identify fractured teeth and teeth with cracks/crazes and bring them to the attention of patient/guardians to avoid being perceived as having "caused a tooth to fracture" after percussing in their child's mouth. A normal percussive response is the absence of pain. Generally, tenderness greater than a contralateral tooth is recorded as "+," and exquisite tenderness is recorded as "++." Overall, this test is based on subjective comparison and is subject to maturity of patient, mental status, and other issues.

Imaging

As far as radiographs are concerned, dedicated dental imaging is of the greatest value. Periapical and occlusal radiographs are best, with panoramic imaging slightly less favorable, especially with the anterior dentition. A panorex machine, however, is more likely to be present in an emergency department and serves as an excellent screening tool for the entire dentition and mandible. Plain skull films may be obtained but generally are of minimal value due to multiple superimposed structures. Three-view CT demonstrates fractures well but significant radiation exposure in children for isolated dentoalveolar injuries may or may not be justifiable.

Lost teeth, fragments, and appliances must be accounted for if not definitively located during physical examination. If concern exists for lost dental debris, chest and/or abdominal imaging is indicated to exclude aspiration or swallowing of debris.

Photography of injuries is useful from a medicolegal perspective and useful for reminding patients/guardians of the pretreatment state of their child's oral cavity.

Antibiotics/Immunizations

Any pediatric injury exposing the pulp tissues, intraoral lacerations, or exposed bone warrants a review of a child's immunization history for tetanus status, and redosing is indicated, as appropriate. It should not be general practice to administer antibiotics for dentoalveolar injuries but may be appropriate in cases of immunosuppression or grossly contaminated wounds.

SPECIFIC INJURY AND TREATMENT

For the sake of simplicity, descriptions of treatment of the primary dentition and permanent dentition are discussed using the Andreasen classification system (**Fig. 7–11**).

Treatment of Injury to the Primary Dentition

Infraction
- Observation, advising patient of fracture and possibility of future worsening and progression of fracture

Uncomplicated enamel limited fracture
- Smooth sharp edges, if possible

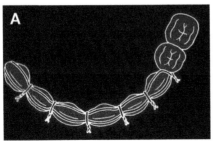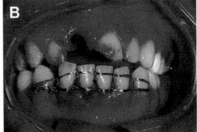

Fig. 7. (A) Essig wire. (B) Essig wire.

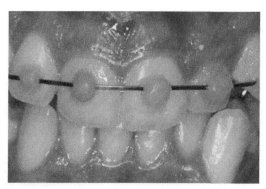

Fig. 8. Flexible composite and orthodontic wire splint.

- Account for tooth fragment
- Refer to general/pediatric dentist for enameloplasty within 2 weeks

Uncomplicated crown fracture

- Seal with glass ionomer cement; do not use zinc oxide eugenol. Refer to general/pediatric dentist for placement of composite and glass ionomer if unavailable within 2 weeks
- Follow-up with general/pediatric dentist 3 to 4 weeks after placement of glass ionomer if done in ED

Complicated crown fracture

- Referral to general/pediatric dentist for partial removal of pulpal tissues and restoration
- If patient unable to see dentist, offer extraction with referral for space maintainer to prevent malocclusion from unilateral extraction

Uncomplicated crown-root fracture

- Removal of tooth fragment only versus extraction
- If tooth fragment removed, perform enameloplasty and refer to pediatric/general dentist for restoration in 2 weeks

Complicated crown-root fracture

- Extract due to poor prognosis of tooth

Root fracture

- If coronal segment is nondisplaced, observe and apply flexible splint for 2 to 4 weeks
- If mobile, extract coronal portion and leave apical portion

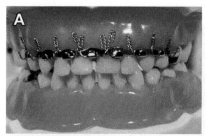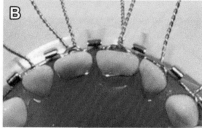

Fig. 9. (*A*) Rigid fixation with arch bars and 24 g wire. (*B*) Additional circumdental wires can be passed over the height of contour to counteract extrusion if encountered with first wires placed under height of contour. Useful with mobile and avulsed dentition but not needed if teeth are very stable in alveolar segment.

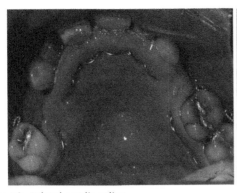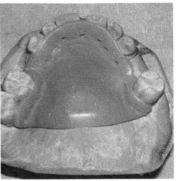

Fig. 10. Palatal acrylic splint.

Concussion
- No need for treatment, observation only
- Soft food for 1 week, good oral hygiene
- Follow-up with general/pediatric dentist in 1 week

Subluxation
- May be no need for treatment
- Apply flexible composite splint with 26–28 g wire or 50 lb test fish line as needed for comfort for 2 weeks
- Soft food for 1 week, good oral hygiene, follow-up with general dentist in 1 week

Extrusion
- For minor extrusion (<3 mm) in immature developing tooth, carefully reposition or leave tooth alone to reposition
- If mature primary tooth or significantly extruded (>3 mm), consider extraction
- No splint required
- Follow-up with general/pediatric dentist in 1 week
- Soft diet, good oral hygiene

Lateral luxation
- Severe labial displacements should be extracted due to high incidence of trauma to permanent developing tooth germ
- If no occlusal interference or not affecting permanent tooth bud (lingual displacements), reposition and place flexible splint for 2 weeks
- Follow-up with general/pediatric dentist in 1 week
- Soft diet, good oral hygiene

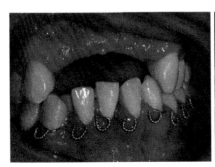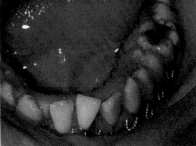

Fig. 11. Lingual splint technique.

Intrusion
- Associated with high incidence of injury to developing permanent tooth bud (advise parents)
- If tooth apex approximates permanent tooth bud, then recommend extraction
- If labially inclined and root exits labial alveolus, allow for spontaneous re-eruption
- Follow-up with general/pediatric dentist in 1 week
- Soft diet, good oral hygiene

Avulsion
- Account for all lost teeth with examination and imaging
- Ensure avulsed tooth is a primary not permanent tooth (likely if under age 6 years)
- *Do not reimplant*
- Follow-up with general/pediatric dentist in 1 week
- Soft diet, good oral hygiene

Injury to the Permanent Dentition

Injury to the permanent dentition follows a similar classification with regard to injury to the hard and soft tissue structures of the dentoalveolar unit. Injury to the permanent dental tissues involves similar treatment to that of the primary dentition. Prompt referral to a general dentist or endodontist is recommended because most necessary materials are not available in an emergency room. Injuries to the permanent dentition with regard to dentoalveolar structures are discussed later. Always consider the caries status and periodontal health of the dentition they are attempting to treat because advanced disease may ultimately result in dentoalveolar injury treatment failure.

Concussion
- No need for treatment, observation only
- Soft food for 1 week, good oral hygiene
- Follow-up with general dentist in 1 week

Subluxation
- May be no need for treatment
- Apply flexible composite splint as needed for comfort for 2 weeks
- Soft food for 1 week, good oral hygiene, follow-up with general dentist in 1 week

Extrusion
- Cleanse area and carefully reposition tooth with axial pressure
- Apply flexible splint for 2 weeks
- Follow-up with general dentist in 1 week
- Soft food for 1 week, good oral hygiene

Lateral luxation
- Cleanse area and carefully reposition tooth with axial pressure
- Apply flexible splint for 2 weeks
- Follow-up with general dentist in approximately 1 week
- Soft food for 1–2 weeks, good oral hygiene

Intrusion
- Associated with a high incidence of tooth loss and tooth resorption
- Dependent on extent of tooth root formation and amount of impaction (see **Table 1**)
- Early endodontic consultation recommended
- Apply flexible splint for 2 weeks

Table 1
Factors determining treatment choice are stages of root development, age, and intrusion level

Degree of Intrusion		Repositioning		
		Spontaneous	Orthodontic	Surgical
Open apex	Up to 7 mm	x	—	—
	More than 7 mm	—	x	x
Closed apex	Up to 3 mm	x	—	—
	3–7 mm	—	x	x
	More than 7 mm	—	—	x

From The dental trauma guide. 2010. Available at: http://www.dentaltraumaguide.org; with permission.

- Follow-up with general dentist in 1 week
- Soft food for 1 to 2 weeks, good oral hygiene

Avulsion

Handle the tooth only by the crown portion and wash under cold water for 10 seconds. Ideal storage media is Hanks balanced salt solution or saline, but placement in the buccal vestibule or milk is suitable. Avoid water or keeping the tooth dry.

Guidelines based on extent of root development and extraoral dry time or transport in nonphysiologic media.

Closed root apex, replanted prior to arrival
- Verify position, apply flexible splint for 2 weeks
- Antibiotic coverage with tetracycline or penicillin for 7 days; ensure tetanus coverage
- Early endodontic consultation recommended
- Follow-up with general dentist in approximately 1 week
- Soft food for 1 to 2 weeks, good oral hygiene

Closed root apex, extraoral dry time or storage in physiologic media for less than 60 minutes
- Clean root surface and irrigate socket with saline
- Reimplant tooth with gentle digital pressure and verify position
- Apply flexible splint for 2 weeks
- Antibiotic coverage with tetracycline or penicillin for 7 days; ensure tetanus coverage
- Early endodontic consultation recommended
- Follow-up with general dentist in approximately 1 week
- Soft food for 1 to 2 weeks, good oral hygiene

Closed root apex, extraoral dry time or storage in physiologic media for greater than 60 minutes
Poor prognosis due to necrosis of the PDL. Goal is to maintain alveolar contour for future dental reconstruction.
- Clean root surface and irrigate socket with saline
- Reimplant tooth with gentle digital pressure and verify position
- Apply flexible splint for 4 weeks
- Antibiotic coverage with tetracycline or penicillin for 7 days; ensure tetanus coverage
- Early endodontic consultation recommended

- Follow-up with general dentist in approximately 1 week
- Soft food for 1–2 weeks, good oral hygiene

Open root apex, replanted prior to arrival
- Verify position, apply flexible splint for 2 weeks
- Antibiotic coverage with tetracycline or penicillin for 7 days; ensure tetanus coverage
- Early endodontic consultation recommended
- Follow-up with general dentist in approximately 1 week
- Soft food for 1 to 2 weeks, good oral hygiene

Open root apex, extraoral dry time or storage in physiologic media for less than 60 minutes
- Clean root surface and irrigate socket with saline
- Topical antibiotics have shown to improve revascularization of dental pulp (minocycline or doxycycline 1 mg per 20 mL saline for 5 minutes soak)
- Reimplant tooth with gentle digital pressure and verify position
- Apply flexible splint for 2 weeks
- Antibiotic coverage with tetracycline or penicillin for 7 days; ensure tetanus coverage
- Early endodontic consultation recommended
- Follow-up with general dentist in approximately 1 week
- Soft food for 1 to 2 weeks, good oral hygiene

Open root apex, extraoral dry time or storage in physiologic media for greater than 60 minutes
   Poor prognosis due to necrosis of the PDL. Goal is to maintain alveolar contour for future dental reconstruction
- Clean root surface and irrigate socket with saline
- Soaking tooth in 2% fluoride solution for 20 minutes shown to decrease rate of osseous resorption
- Reimplant tooth with gentle digital pressure and verify position
- Apply flexible splint for 4 weeks
- Antibiotic coverage with tetracycline or penicillin for 7 days; ensure tetanus coverage
- Early endodontic consultation recommended. Follow-up with general dentist in approximately 1 week

TREATMENT OF INJURIES TO THE SUPPORTING DENTOALVEOLAR BONE

Injury to the supporting alveolar bone often exists in combination with injuries (discussed previously); thus, treatment is often geared toward treating both injuries (**Fig. 12**). Treatment of injuries to alveolar bone in isolation is discussed. This often presents as a segment of teeth (usually 2–3) that has been displaced as a unit in one direction, with the involved teeth not independently mobile.

   Fracture of both alveolar cortices
- Generally poorest prognosis of alveolar fractures but most common due to high incidence of combined dentoalveolar injuries. Often involves comminution of at least one cortex.
- Avoid performing full-thickness mucoperiosteal flaps that may devitalize bone fragments.

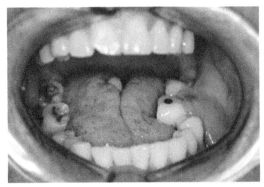

Fig. 12. Nonreduced dentoalveolar fracture of the left posterior mandible interfering with occlusion.

- Apply rigid splinting for 4 to 6 weeks with Erich arch bars, Essig wire, composite retained splints with 24-g wire or acrylic splints that are wired in place. The stabilized segment should extend at least to 2 solid teeth on either side of the mobile teeth.
- Follow-up with general/pediatric dentist in 1 week
- Soft diet, good oral hygiene

Fracture of a single cortex
- Same as for comminution of both cortices but generally with better prognosis
- Patient requires rigid fixation for 4–6 weeks
- Follow-up the general/pediatric dentist in 1 week
- Soft diet, good oral hygiene

Mandible or maxillary fracture

Treatment is beyond the scope of this discussion. It is common to have dentoalveolar fractures with fracture of the mandible and maxilla that is subtle and interferes with obtaining ideal intermaxillary fixation.

SUMMARY

Dentoalveolar trauma is seen by all individuals treating facial trauma. Although the long-term follow-up of the dentition may lie beyond the scope of facial trauma surgeons, important steps can be taken to improve dentoalveolar structure prognosis and treatment outcome. The intent of this article is to provide an overview of treatment of dental injuries as encountered in an emergency department. Timely referral to a general/pediatric dentist or endodontist is appropriate in almost all cases. Consultation with an oral and maxillofacial surgeon is also indicated for immediate treatment as well as for a discussion centered on dental implant reconstruction of the area, should it be required.

REFERENCES

1. Norton NS. Netter's head and neck anatomy for dentistry. 2nd edition. Philadelphia: Elsevier Saunders; 2012.
2. Andreasen JO, Andreasen FM. Textbook and color atlas of traumatic injuries to the teeth. 4th edition. St Louis (MO): Mosby; 2007.

3. Fountain SB, Camp JH. Traumatic injuries. In: Cohen S, Burns RC, editors. Pathways of the pulp. 8th edition. St Louis (MO): Mosby; 2002.
4. Bell WH. Le Forte I osteotomy for correction of maxillary deformities. J Oral Surg 1975;33:412.
5. Glendor U. Epidemiology of traumatic dental injuries–a 12 year review of the literature. Dent Traumatol 2008;24(6).
6. Dental trauma guide. 2010. Available at: http://www.dentaltraumaguide.org.
7. Andreasen JO. Classification, etiology and epidemiology. In: Andreases JO, editor. Traumatic injuries to teeth. 2nd edition. Copenhagen (Denmark): Munksgaard; 1981.
8. U.S Department of Health and Human Services, Children Bureau. National child abuse and neglect system. Summary of key findings from calendar year 2000. 2002. Available at: http://www.acf.hhs.gov/news/press/2002/abuse.html.
9. Laskin DM. The recognition of child abuse. J Oral Surg 1978;36:349.
10. Davidoff G, Jakubowski M, Thomas D, et al. The spectrum of closed-head injury in the facial trauma victims: incidence and impact. Ann Emerg Med 1988;17:27.
11. Holan G, McTigue D. Introduction to dental trauma: managing traumatic injuries in the primary dentition. In: Pinkham JR, Casamassimo PS, Fields HW Jr, et al, editors. Pediatric dentistry: infancy through adolescence. 4th edition. St Louis (MO): Elselvier Sunders; 2005. p. 236–56.
12. Ravn JJ. Sequelae of acute mechanical trauma in the primary dentition. J Dent Child 1968;35(4):281–9.
13. Ravn JJ. Follow-up study of permanent incisiors with enamel cracks as a result or acute trauma. Scand J Dent Res 1981;89(2):117–23.

Soft Tissue Facial Trauma

Traumatic Facial Nerve Injury

Linda N. Lee, MD, Sofia Lyford-Pike, MD, Kofi Derek O. Boahene, MD*

KEYWORDS

- Facial paralysis • Facial nerve injury • Reanimation

KEY POINTS

- If the facial nerve is anatomically intact, or if the injury is limited to the medial portion of a peripheral branch, treatment is usually medical with close observation and possible electrophysiologic testing for monitoring of progression.
- If the nerve is transected, immediate exploration with direct anastamosis provides the best chance of recovery.
- If a large segment of nerve is injured, an interposition graft should be placed immediately. If the injured segment is not easily accessible for repair, nerve transposition is the treatment of choice.
- For facial muscles with irreparable damage or extensive disuse atrophy, muscle transfer procedures are the best option for dynamic facial reanimation.
- Regardless of the type of injury or treatment, ocular protection is of primary concern to prevent avoidable complications.
- Treatment of traumatic facial nerve injuries can be a variable and dynamic process, but having a clear understanding of the diagnostic and treatment algorithms can help of a meaningful recovery for these patients.

INTRODUCTION

Trauma to the facial nerve is the second most common cause of facial paralysis and can result in devastating consequences including ocular complications, impaired speech, feeding difficulties, and inability to convey emotion through facial expression. It is critical that otolaryngologists and facial plastic surgeons have a thorough understanding of the principles of facial nerve trauma management because timing of treatment can have a significant impact on a patient's chances and extent of recovery. The number of possible treatment options can be overwhelming to both patient and physician, including whether or not surgery is indicated and, if so, which operation should be chosen and at what point in time should it be performed.

Department of Otolaryngology Head and Neck Surgery, 601 North Caroline Street, 6th Floor, Johns Hopkins Outpatient Center, Baltimore, MD 21287, USA
* Corresponding author.
E-mail address: dboahen1@jhmi.edu

Otolaryngol Clin N Am 46 (2013) 825–839
http://dx.doi.org/10.1016/j.otc.2013.07.001
0030-6665/13/$ – see front matter © 2013 Elsevier Inc. All rights reserved.

EVALUATION

Management of traumatic facial nerve injuries depends on the timing of facial paralysis after trauma (immediate vs delayed), the extent of paralysis (complete vs incomplete), the type of trauma (blunt, penetrating, or iatrogenic), the condition of the nerve, the duration of facial paralysis, and the status of the motor end plates of the facial muscles.

One key factor that should be assessed in all cases is the potential for recovery of facial function. Reversibility of facial function depends on both the integrity of the nerve and the status of the end-organ facial muscles. In general, if the motor end plates of the facial muscles are still functional, treatment should be aimed at restoring innervation to the facial muscle. If the motor end plates are not functional, then treatment should be focused on transferring an alternate muscle to restore dynamic facial movement.

Details from the history, pertinent clinical examination, neuroimaging, and facial nerve testing can provide the necessary data to guide the decision-making process. A treatment algorithm is presented to help physicians simplify the management strategy and maximize the chances of optimal facial nerve recovery (**Fig. 1**).

Critical questions in the decision tree include
1. Is the facial muscle function reversible (ie, are the motor end plates intact)?
2. Is the facial nerve interrupted or anatomically intact?
3. Is the facial weakness complete or incomplete?
4. Was the onset of paralysis immediate or delayed?
5. Is the injury medial or lateral to the lateral canthus?
6. Is the location of facial nerve injury surgically accessible?
7. Are the facial muscles irreparably damaged, either through direct trauma or atrophy from chronic denervation?
8. Is electrophysiologic testing useful given the time frame?

ANATOMY

The injured segment of the facial nerve can be classified according to its location: intracranial, intratemporal, or extratemporal. The intracranial component of the nerve runs from its origin at the ventral aspect of the pontomedullary junction of the brain stem to the porus acousticus of the internal auditory canal (IAC). The intratemporal component includes the portion of the nerve from within the IAC to the stylomastoid foramen and is subdivided to include the meatal, labyrinthine, tympanic (horizontal), and mastoid (vertical) segments. The tympanic segment is dehiscent in 40% to 50% of people, and is therefore the most commonly injured segment during middle ear and mastoid surgery. The extratemporal nerve then begins at the level of the stylomastoid foramen and ends at the motor end plates of the muscles of facial expression. After exiting the stylomastoid foramen, the extratemporal facial nerve divides at the main pes anserine into the temporofacial and cervicofacial branches. These 2 branches then further divide into the temporal, zygomatic, buccal, marginal mandibular, and cervical branches. All muscles of facial expression are innervated on their deep surface except for the mentalis, levator anguli oris, and buccinator muscles.[1]

CAUSES OF FACIAL NERVE TRAUMA

Facial nerve injury can be a result of blunt or penetrating trauma. The most common cause of facial nerve injury is blunt trauma from a fracture of the temporal bone.[1,2] Motor vehicle accidents are also common sources of blunt trauma that can damage

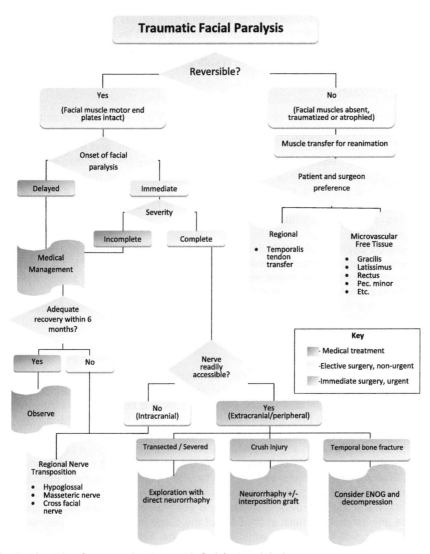

Fig. 1. Algorithm for managing traumatic facial nerve injuries.

the facial nerve. Typical examples of penetrating trauma that may produce facial nerve injury include animal bites to the face, laceration from knife trauma, or blast injuries from gunshot wounds, explosives, or slag injury.

Injuries to the facial nerve can also occur iatrogenically and arise most frequently during salivary gland and otologic surgeries. Traumatic forceps delivery during birth can result in injury to the facial nerve of the newborn.

CLASSIFICATION OF NERVE DAMAGE

The severity of gross damage to the nerve varies and can include simple traction injury with an anatomically intact nerve, crush injury, partial or full transection, or loss of a segment of nerve. The extent of nerve damage can help predict recovery. In general, nerve injuries that result in disruption of the neural tube require surgical intervention for recovery. In 1943, Seddon classified nerve damage into 3 levels (**Table 1**).[3]

In 1951, Sunderland then further divided the Seddon III Neurotmesis category based on the level of the neural tube affected (**Table 2**).[4]

INITIAL ASSESSMENT

Cases of trauma to the face, head, and neck, as with all cases of significant trauma, should begin with a primary survey assessing the patient's airway, breathing, and circulation. Wounds should be cleaned and copiously irrigated, and antibiotic therapy and any necessary tetanus prophylaxis should be administered. Detailed examination of facial movement can then be performed, including eyebrow movement, eye closure with gentle and full effort, midface movement, and capacity to smile and pucker. If possible, any sedation should be lightened for the facial nerve examination. If the patient is unable to cooperate, a transient noxious stimuli can be used to assess for a grimace.

If facial paralysis is noted to be incomplete or segmental, a thorough description of the involved branches and the severity of paresis/paralysis is helpful to accompany a grade from an established facial nerve grading system. A video or a series of photographs can be helpful to document the baseline clinical examination. If the patient is noted to have complete facial paralysis, an effort should be made to determine whether this paralysis is of immediate or delayed onset.

ELECTROPHYSIOLOGIC TESTING

Electroneuronography (ENOG) and electromyography (EMG) are 2 electrodiagnostic tests that can aid in the clinical decision making when considering whether to intervene in a traumatic facial nerve injury. If the facial nerve is believed to be anatomically intact, these tests can help determine whether the injury is a Sunderland I or II, or whether the injury is more severe.[4] Electrophysiologic testing is not needed in incomplete facial paralysis or in segmental paralysis. In cases of complete paralysis, these tests are not helpful in the first 3 days after injury, because, even in a fully transected nerve, Wallerian degeneration has not had time to occur and the nerve continues to transmit distal impulses and potentially provide a false-positive result.[5] ENOG uses a surface electrode to provide stimulation to the main trunk of the facial nerve and records any action potentials at the level of the distal facial muscles. The response on the paretic side is compared with the normal side. ENOG can be tested in a serial fashion, and if more than 90% degeneration is seen compared with the normal side, surgical intervention can be considered.[6–8]

In practice, it is logistically difficult to see patients with traumatic facial paralysis in the early period and perform serial ENOG in the critical 6 days after facial paralysis. This may partly be due to limited availability of electrodiagnostic resources or the

Table 1	
Seddon's 1943 classification of nerve damage	
I. Neuropraxia	Conduction block only
II. Axonotmesis	Wallerian degeneration occurs but axonal contents are intact
III. Neurotmesis	Axon is disrupted Surgical intervention likely required for recovery Synkinesis likely to develop

Table 2
Sunderland's modification of Seddon's nerve damage classification

I. Neuropraxia	Conduction block only No Wallerian degeneration Full spontaneous recovery expected
II. Axonotmesis	Wallerian degeneration occurs but axonal contents are intact Full spontaneous recovery expected (neural regeneration rate of ~1 mm/d)
III. Neurotmesis Type II + endoneural injury	Surgical intervention likely required for recovery
IV. Neurotmesis Type III + perineural injury	Surgical intervention likely required for recovery
V. Neurotmesis Type IV + epineural injury	Surgical intervention likely required for recovery

presence of other more serious injuries. At 2 to 3 weeks after an injury resulting in complete facial paralysis, EMG is the most helpful electrophysiologic test to determine whether the nerve is in the process of recovery. Myogenic electrical activity is recorded with a needle inserted into the end-organ facial muscle. The presence of fibrillation potentials indicates nerve degeneration, whereas polyphasic action potentials indicate neural regeneration.[7,8]

RADIOGRAPHIC IMAGING

In cases of complete facial paralysis in patients with trauma to the skull, high-resolution computed tomography (CT) with fine cuts (1-mm slices) through the temporal bone can be useful to evaluate for disruption of the fallopian canal. Contrast is generally not needed unless there is concern about associated vascular injury. When gross fracture lines are not obvious, the region around the geniculate ganglion fossa (GGF) should be closely inspected. An enlarged GGF on temporal bone CT is an additional clue for the diagnosis of GGF fracture in patients with traumatic facial paralysis. This correlates with findings of edema, fibrosis, bony spicules impinging on the facial nerve often found in the GGF when decompressing the facial nerve in cases of trauma.

MANAGEMENT

An approach to treating trauma-related facial nerve injuries is to categorize the injuries into reversible and irreversible palsies. Patients with injuries that are considered reversible have viable and functional facial muscles, and treatment is aimed at reinnervation of these muscles through repair of the facial nerve or transposing another nerve to power the distal end of the facial nerve. Patients without viable facial muscles have irreversible injuries and typically require functional muscle transfers to restore facial movement. Static slings and suspension procedures can be considered as adjuvant interventions to further improve symmetry and function.

Reversible Facial Nerve Injury

The primary consideration in the initial management of a patient with a traumatic facial paralysis is the reversibility of facial muscle function. In cases of reversible injury, it is important to determine which cases will recover spontaneously with medical therapy and close observation and which warrant immediate surgical repair. Answering the following questions help to clarify the next step to take:

1. Was the onset of facial weakness immediate or delayed?
2. If the onset was immediate, is the facial weakness complete, incomplete?
3. If the onset is immediate and the paralysis is complete, is the damaged segment located medially or laterally to the lateral canthus of the eye?
4. In complete paralysis, is the nerve anatomically continuous or interrupted?
5. When the nerve is interrupted, can the proximal segment be easily mobilized for nerve grafting?

Medical treatment and expectant observation

Medical therapy and close observation is appropriate for those patients with incomplete paralysis, delayed onset of paralysis, blunt trauma to the extratemporal nerve, and injury that occurs medial to the lateral canthus of the eye. In these categories of patients, recovery is usually spontaneous without the need for immediate surgical exploration or repair. Some traumatic birth injuries resolve spontaneously and without surgical intervention. If medical therapy is chosen, the patient should be closely observed to ensure that a meaningful and sufficient recovery is achieved in a timely manner. If sufficient recovery is not evident within 6 months after the trauma, surgical intervention should then be considered to prevent irreversible chronic atrophy of the facial muscles (typically with a nerve transposition procedure).

Cases of incomplete paralysis secondary to injury or edema are associated with a nerve that is anatomically continuous with neuropraxia or axonotmesis. Treatment should be aimed at minimizing edema and preventing viral infection. The use of steroids is supported in the treatment of incomplete paralysis,[9,10] but there are mixed data on the benefit of antivirals.[11]

Delayed onset of complete or incomplete paralysis suggests an anatomically intact nerve, with delayed neuropraxia or axonotmesis. This diagnosis requires certainty that facial function was transiently intact immediately after the injury, either from direct examination or by obtaining a clear history from the initial trauma team or family members. In cases of delayed complete paralysis, some investigators recommend serial electrophysiologic testing with ENOG between days 3 and 14, and consideration of surgical facial nerve decompression if there is greater than 95% loss of axonal function compared with the unaffected side.[6] In cases of possible iatrogenic injury, it is important to determine if the nerve was noted to be anatomically intact and stimulated at the end of the procedure. Adequate time should also be allowed for the effect of local anesthetic to wear off to account for cases of temporary paresis from medication. Initial treatment with steroids to minimize inflammation and edema is reasonable.

Blunt trauma to the extratemporal nerve is usually managed conservatively with expectant observation. Surgery is considered if no recovery is seen after 6 months.

Injury that occurs medial to the lateral canthus of the eye rarely results in clinical paralysis. In the midface, there are rich cross-anastomotic connections of the nerve that allow spontaneous recovery of facial function.[7,8] However, in the rare circumstance that an injury medial to the lateral canthus does cause clinical paralysis of that segment, then exploration of the nerve with repair should be considered.

Traumatic birth injuries are usually associated with emergency forceps delivery. Because the stylomastoid foramen is more lateralized in infants compared with adults, the main trunk of the nerve is at high risk for external trauma. Fortunately, more than 90% of traumatic birth injuries to the facial nerve resolve spontaneously without long-term sequelae.[12]

Early surgical exploration and repair

When traumatic injury to the face and head results in immediate paralysis, it should be assumed that the facial nerve is interrupted or severely crushed to result in neurotmesis. Early surgical exploration and repair is indicated for such patients (**Fig. 2**). The ease of exploration and the approach selected depends on the suspected site of injury. Exploration within 3 days of injuries allows the use of a nerve stimulator to identify distal segments of disrupted facial nerve branches. If there are contraindications to immediate repair, then efforts should be made to tag the nerve endings for easier identification during a subsequent staged repair.

To determine the ideal surgical repair of the nerve, the following questions should be addressed:

1. Is the facial nerve proximal to the injury accessible? Although intracranial injuries are not easily accessible, extracranial injuries can be more readily explored.
2. Can a direct neurorrhaphy be performed without excessive tension on the anastamosis (ie, is the nerve simply transected or is there a segment of nerve that is injured or missing)?
3. If the injury is iatrogenic, was the nerve directly visualized during surgery?

If the damaged portion of the nerve is extracranial (eg, temporal bone fracture or injury to the intraparotid nerve), then the best outcomes are achieved with direct nerve repair. If the nerve is transected, end-to-end neurorrhaphy with microscope-assisted anastamosis provides the best chance of recovery. Various techniques for coapting nerves have been studied including epineural sutures, perineural sutures, and sutureless fibrin glue coaptation. A tension-free repair that maximizes alignment of neural axons is more important than the technique chosen. The nerve can be mobilized to allow direct neurorrhaphy in defects less than 2 cm. Excessive mobilization of the nerve should be avoided to prevent devascularization.

If a segment of severe crush injury needs to be resected or if there is a missing segment of nerve, an interposition nerve graft or neural conduit should be placed to bridge the segments and to prevent tension on the anastomoses. The most frequently used donor nerve grafts include the sural nerve, great auricular nerve, and the medial antebrachial cutaneous nerve. These sensory nerve grafts are associated with minimal donor site morbidity that is generally well tolerated. Sural nerve grafts can provide the most length (up to 35 cm).[13,14] Motor nerve allografts up to 7 cm in length are now commercially available and can be used instead of donor nerves.

In cases of temporal bone fractures with immediate facial nerve paralysis, surgical exploration with nerve decompression, removal of any penetrating bony fragments, and neurorrhaphy of interrupted segments should be performed. Longitudinal fractures involving the IAC is best explored with a middle cranial fossa approach.

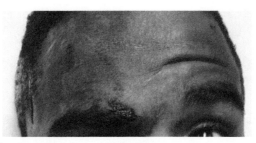

Fig. 2. Immediate facial paralysis from a stab injury.

Fractures of the vertical segment of the facial nerve are explored with a transmastoid approach. Mixed fractures may require both approaches.

In cases of iatrogenic injury with immediate onset of complete paralysis, the surgeon should be asked about the details of the case. If the nerve was not directly visualized or the surgeon is not confident about the integrity of the nerve, then reexploration should be performed after enough time has passed for any local anesthetic to be metabolized. Given the inherent emotional distress associated with iatrogenic facial nerve injury, surgeons are advised to consider consulting a colleague to help with the nerve exploration.

In cases of iatrogenic injury with gradual onset or incomplete paralysis, the patient should be closely monitored for progression. Electrophysiologic testing should be considered if the paralysis becomes complete. The decision to reexplore depends on what is believed to be the cause of trauma. If an exposed nerve is believed to be compressed by a bony spicule, graft or implant, prompt reexploration to relieve the compression is necessary once progressive weakness is documented. If the trauma was from traction, recovery without surgical intervention is more likely.

In cases of intracranial injury to the nerve, an interposition graft from the proximal portion of the nerve in the brain stem to the distal uninjured nerve can be performed at the time of injury. A delayed craniotomy for access to an injured facial nerve in the IAC is feasible but the inherent risks of such a procedure should be carefully weighed against the potential benefits before proceeding. In cases of reversible paralysis when the proximal facial nerve is not available, a regional cranial motor nerve can be recruited to reinnervate the paralyzed facial muscles. Commonly recruited cranial nerves include the contralateral facial nerve, the hypoglossal, and the masseter nerve. Historically, the spinal accessory nerve has been used for crossover grafting, but this nerve has largely fallen out of favor secondary to the morbidity of trapezius muscle atrophy and the inferior facial movement results compared with using the hypoglossal and masseteric nerves. However, the identification and use of the sternocleidomastoid branch of the accessory nerve, while preserving motor innervation to the trapezius, has been described. The spinal accessory nerve is still a viable option for nerve transposition if the hypoglossal or masseteric nerves are not available.[15,16]

The hypoglossal nerve has been widely used to reinnervate the facial muscle. Various techniques have been described including an interposition graft between the facial and hypoglossal nerves, complete transection and translocation of the hypoglossal nerve to the facial nerve, and translocation of the intratemporal facial nerve to the hypoglossal nerve (**Fig. 3**).

The axonal density of the masseteric nerve contributes to its high success rate in facial nerve reanimation cases.[17,18] Another advantage of the masseteric branch as a regional transfer is its proximity to the facial nerve. The length and proximity allow

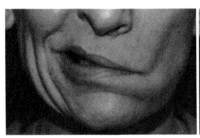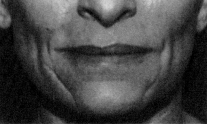

Fig. 3. Facial to hypoglossal nerve transfer result.

for the transposition and anastomosis of the nerves without the need for an interposition graft.[17,18] The subzygomatic triangle recently described by Collar and colleagues[15] is a reliable anatomic landmark for identifying and mobilizing the master nerve for facial reanimation (**Fig. 4**).

Irreversible Facial Nerve Injury

Traumatic facial nerve injury is deemed irreversible when the motor end plates are nonfunctional. This can be due to chronic denervation to the muscle resulting in irreversible muscle atrophy, or trauma that results in a significant loss of muscle tissue (eg, blast or gunshot injury, or animal bite). In these cases, reestablishing dynamic facial movement requires replacing the native facial muscles with a new functional muscle.

Dynamic muscle transfer techniques include regional muscle transfer, regional muscle tendon unit transfer (eg., temporalis tendon transfer), and microvascular free functional muscle transfer (gracilis, latissimus, rectus, pectoralis, or others). For patients with irreversible facial nerve injury who are not candidates for dynamic muscle transfer, static slings with fascia lata or synthetic materials are an option for providing some improvement in facial symmetry.

Muscle tendon unit transfer

Temporalis tendon transfer can be performed in an orthodromic, minimally invasive fashion using either a 2-cm incision in the nasolabial fold or a completely intraoral approach.[19,20] To optimize the dynamic motion of the oral commissure, the length-tension relationship of the tendon should be analyzed intraoperatively (**Fig. 5**). Problems with excessive or inadequate tension on the tendon can result in suboptimal muscle contraction.[21,22]

Free functional muscle transfer

The gracilis muscle is the most commonly used free tissue transfer for dynamic facial reanimation (**Fig. 6**). It can be performed as a single-stage procedure driven by the masseteric branch of the trigeminal nerve or as a 2-stage procedure driven by the contralateral cross-facial nerve graft. The 2-stage procedure has the benefit of allowing a spontaneous mimetic smile. In the first stage of the procedure, the sural nerve graft is anastomosed to a buccal branch of the intact contralateral facial nerve and tunneled into the cutaneous upper lip on the paralyzed side. The second stage is performed when tapping on the distal end of the cross-face sural nerve graft produces tingling

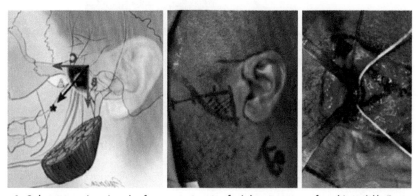

Fig. 4. Subzygomatic triangle for masseter to facial nerve transfer. (*Asterisk*) Expected course of masseter nerve; (B) anterior border of temporomandibular joint; (C) Inferior border of zygomatic arch.

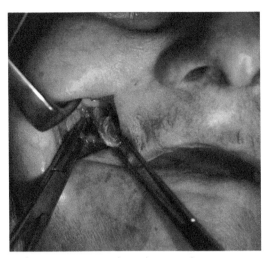

Fig. 5. Temporalis tendon exposure, transbuccal approach.

on the intact side (Tinel sign).[10,23,24] The timing of the second stage can vary but usually occurs 6 to 12 months after the first stage. The gracilis muscle can also be innervated using both the masseter and cross-facial nerve grafts for a more predictable result.

In cases of an open wound from a blast injury or animal bite that results in significant loss of muscle tissue, immediate attention is paid to wound care, including debridement and washout and appropriate antibiotics to prevent infection. Once the wound is stabilized, muscle transfer techniques can be considered in a staged fashion.

For patients who are not candidates for muscle transfer or microvascular free flaps, static slings are an option for improving facial symmetry. Slings can be autologous material (eg, fascia lata) or synthetic (eg, Gortex), depending on patient and surgeon preference.[7,8]

OCULAR PROTECTION

For all patients with facial paralysis, appropriate eye care is paramount to prevent corneal dryness and infection, which can ultimately lead to permanent vision loss.

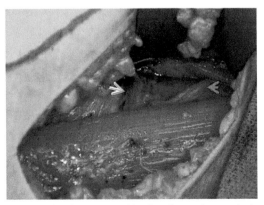

Fig. 6. Gracilis muscle transfer for irreversible facial muscle paralysis. *White arrowhead* shows the vascular pedicle to gracilis muscle and the *blue arrowhead* shows the obturator nerve to gracilis muscle.

The most commonly used conservative therapies include artificial tears, ophthalmic ointments, moisture chambers, and protective eye taping. Chemodenervation of the levator palpebral superioris or Mueller muscle can also be performed.

In the assessment of ocular risk in patients with paralytic lagophthalmos and/or ectropion, the following 4 aspects of the eye examination should be routinely evaluated and documented[23]:

1. Is there a positive Bell phenomenon?
2. Is corneal sensation intact? (test with cotton wisp)
3. Are there problems with dry eye? (The Shirmer test can be considered. Diminished tearing and loss of corneal sensation can be sequelae of trigeminal injury that increase the risk of ocular complications.)

Patients with corneal hypesthesia, severe lagophthalmos, and absent Bell phenomenon are at the highest risk for corneal desiccation and subsequent exposure keratopathy and infection. Aggressive lubrication, close monitoring with routine ocular examinations, and early surgical intervention with lid loading and/or lower eyelid tightening procedures should be considered in these patients. A tarsorrhaphy should may considered in patients with severe lagophthalmos and corneal anesthesia.[23]

Upper Eyelid Loading

Surgical management of the paralytic eyelid includes static loading with platinum or gold weights placed over the tarsal plate. The size of the weight is determined by taping different sized weights to the upper lid 2 mm above the lash line. The sizing is determined with the patient in the upright position, and the smallest weight that provides eye closure with gentle effort is chosen. If the weight is too heavy, mechanical ptosis can cause visual field obstruction. An incision is made in the supratarsal crease and dissection is carried down to the tarsal plate. A pocket is dissected over the tarsal plate centered just medial to the pupil. The weight is secured to the tarsal plate using 3 sutures and the orbicularis and skin are reapproximated. Historically, gold weights have been used, but platinum weights may be advantageous given their lower profile and reduced rate of extrusion and capsule formation compared with gold weights.[23] Eyelid weights can be removed if facial nerve function recovers.

Lower Eyelid Repositioning

If lower eyelid paralytic ectropion is present, lower lid tightening procedures can be performed. These include spacer grafts, lateral transorbital canthopexy (which does not shorten the horizontal aperture), lateral tarsal strip (which shortens the horizontal aperture), and medial canthopexy via a transcutaneous, transcaruncular, or precaruncular approach.[25] The goal of medial canthopexy is to reapproximate the inferior punctum against the globe to prevent buildup of tears in the sulcus. Patients should be assessed for a negative vector eye, where the anterior-most portion of the globe is positioned anterior to the orbital rim. In this select group of patients, ectropion is not easily repaired by typical canthopexy or canthoplasty procedures; traditional lower eyelid procedures can worsen eyelid malposition if not recognized preoperatively. Midface lifting procedures can be considered to help with ectropion in this group.[23]

ADJUNCT TREATMENT/OPTIONS FOR IMPROVING FACIAL ASYMMETRY

Supplemental techniques that can help to provide immediate improvement in facial symmetry while awaiting facial nerve recovery can be of particular benefit to patients presenting with facial nerve trauma of chronic duration. Brow lifts can be performed for paralytic brow ptosis, and midface or full facelifts can help improve facial symmetry. Autologous fat augmentation can improve midface atrophy, which can lead to improved cosmesis and patient confidence. These complementary procedures can be performed unilaterally or bilaterally depending on the patient's needs and desires. With advance planning, these techniques can often be done simultaneously during the facial nerve exploration and reinnervation operation.[23,25]

For patients with long-standing facial nerve trauma who develop synkinesis, selective and directed chemodenervation can control synkinesis. Platysmectomy can be considered as a more permanent treatment for patients with good response to chemodenervation of platysmal banding and spasm.[26]

PHYSICAL THERAPY

Physical therapy and nonsurgical rehabilitation methods play a significant role in treatment and recovery of facial paralysis. These techniques may be used as a primary modality or as an adjunct to the therapies described earlier.[27] Physical therapy focused on neuromuscular retraining can be effective in lessening the sequelae of aberrant facial reinnervation. The goals of neuromuscular retraining therapy are to minimize the undesirable synkinetic movement and hypercontracture while enhancing the desired movement of the recovering facial muscles.

Facets of facial physical therapy treatment can include[28,29]

- Patient education
- Relaxation training
- Face-tapping exercises
- Behavioral training with biofeedback (visual or EMG sensory feedback)
- Specific action exercises
- Stress integration and voice patterning
- Eyelid-specific action exercises
- Electrical stimulation
- Mechanical/manual stimulation or massage
- Facial strengthening exercises

Most commonly, treatment comprises facial neuromuscular retraining exercises with or without visual or EMG biofeedback, mechanical or manual stimulation, and/or electrical stimulation. Neuromuscular retraining has shown efficacy in restoring function in long-standing facial paralysis.[28,30] A randomized controlled trial in 2007 supported an individually tailored facial neuromuscular training program in patients with Bell palsy.[31] The inclusion of biofeedback, either through visual feedback or EMG, reduces recovery times, improves facial symmetry, and reduces synkinesis.[32,33] A randomized controlled trial demonstrated no difference between visual feedback or EMG.[34] Several studies on a rat facial paralysis model show benefit from mechanical stimulation.[35–37] Mechanical stimulation in the form of massage is often used in conjunction with neuromuscular retraining.

Cai and colleagues[38] evaluated the efficacy of functional training of mimic muscles in incomplete facial nerve injury. A total of 241 injured facial nerve branches were evaluated with follow-up at 1 and 4 years. All patients (both treatment and control) received treatment with vitamin B_{12}, vitamin B_1, and electrical stimulation. The paradigm for the treatment group included massage (2–4 times per day) and exercises for specific facial muscle groups. In patients with moderate to severe deficits (House-Brackmann scores III to VI), inclusion of exercises and therapy improved recovery rates and reduced synkinesis and hemifacial spasm.[38] No benefit was found for patients with minor (House-Brackmann II) deficits.

SUMMARY

Facial nerve trauma can be a devastating injury resulting in functional deficits and psychological distress. Deciding on the optimal course of treatment for patients with traumatic facial nerve injuries can be challenging, as there are many critical factors to be considered for each patient.[39] Choosing from the great array of therapeutic options available can become overwhelming to both patients and physicians, and in this article, the authors present a systematic approach to help organize the physician's thought process.

If the nerve is anatomically intact or if the injury is limited to the medial portion of a peripheral branch, treatment is usually medical with close observation and possible electrophysiologic testing for monitoring of progression. If the nerve is transected, immediate exploration with direct anastamosis provides the best chance of recovery. If a large segment of nerve is injured, an interposition graft should be placed immediately. If the injured segment is not easily accessible for repair, nerve transposition is the treatment of choice. For facial muscles with irreparable damaged or extensive disuse atrophy, muscle transfer procedures are the best option for dynamic facial reanimation.

Regardless of the type of injury or treatment chosen, ocular protection should be of primary concern to prevent avoidable complications. The treatment of traumatic facial nerve injuries can be a variable and dynamic process, but having a clear understanding of the diagnostic and treatment algorithms can help maximize the chances of a meaningful recovery for these patients.

REFERENCES

1. May M. Anatomy for the clinician. In: May M, Schaitkin B, editors. The facial nerve. New York: Thieme Medical Publishers; 2000. p. 19–56.
2. Chang CY, Cass SP. Management of facial nerve injury due to temporal bone trauma. Am J Otol 1999;20:96–114.
3. Seddon HJ. A classification of nerve injuries. Br Med J 1942;29:237–9.
4. Sunderland S. The anatomy and physiology of nerve injury. Muscle Nerve 1990; 13:771–84.
5. Sittel C, Stennert E. Prognostic value of electromyography in acute peripheral facial nerve palsy. Otol Neurotol 2001;22:100–4.
6. Gantz BJ, Rubinstein JT, Gidley P, et al. Surgical management of Bell's palsy. Laryngoscope 1999;109:1177–88.
7. Coker NJ. Acute paralysis of the facial nerve. In: Bailey BJ, editor. Head and neck surgery – otolaryngology. Philadelphia: J.B. Lippincott; 1993. p. 1711–28.
8. Clark JM, Shockley WW. Management and reanimation of the paralyzed face. In: Papel ID, editor. Facial plastic and reconstructive surgery. New York: Thieme Medical Publishers; 2002. p. 660–85.
9. Salinas RA, Alvarez G, Daly F, et al. Corticosteroids for Bell's palsy (idiopathic facial paralysis). Cochrane Database Syst Rev 2010;(3):CD001942.
10. Hadlock T. Facial paralysis: research and future directions. Facial Plast Surg 2008;24:260–7.
11. Lockhart P, Daly F, Pitkethly M, et al. Antiviral treatment for Bell's palsy (idiopathic facial paralysis). Cochrane Database Syst Rev 2009;(4):CD001869.

12. Smith JD, Crumley RL, Harker LA. Facial paralysis in the newborn. Otolaryngol Head Neck Surg 1981;89:336–42.
13. Humphrey CD, Kriet JD. Nerve repair and cable grafting for facial paralysis. Facial Plast Surg 2008;24:170–6.
14. Conley J, Baker DC. Hypoglossal-facial nerve anastamosis for reinnervation of the paralyzed face. Plast Reconstr Surg 1979;63:63–72.
15. Collar RM, Byrne PJ, Boahene KD. The subzygomatic triangle: rapid, minimally invasive identification of the masseteric nerve for facial reanimation. Plast Reconstr Surg 2013;132(1):183–8.
16. Poe DS, Scher N, Panje WR. Facial reanimation by XI-VII anastamosis without shoulder paralysis. Laryngoscope 1989;99:1040–7.
17. Coombs CJ, Ek EW, Wu T, et al. Masseteric-facial nerve coaptation – an alternative technique for facial nerve reanimation. J Plast Reconstr Aesthet Surg 2009; 62:1580–8.
18. Borschel GH, Kawamura DH, Kasukurthi R, et al. The motor nerve to the masseter muscle: an anatomic and histomorphometric study to facilitate its use in facial reanimation. J Plast Reconstr Aesthet Surg 2012;65:363–6.
19. Boahene KD, Farrag TY, Ishii L, et al. Minimally invasive temporalis tendon transposition. Arch Facial Plast Surg 2011;13:8–13.
20. Byrne PJ, Kim M, Boahene K, et al. Temporalis tendon transfer as part of a comprehensive approach to facial reanimation. Arch Facial Plast Surg 2007;9: 234–41.
21. Boahene KD. Principles and biomechanics of muscle tendon unit transfer: application in temporalis muscle tendon transposition for smile improvement in facial paralysis. Laryngoscope 2013;123(2):350–5.
22. Bae YC, Zuker RM, Manktelow RT, et al. A comparison of commissure excursion following gracilis muscle transplantation for facial paralysis using a cross-face nerve graft versus the motor nerve to the masseteric nerve. Plast Reconstr Surg 2006;117:2407–13.
23. Chan JY, Byrne PJ. Management of facial paralysis in the 21st century. Facial Plast Surg 2011;27:346–57.
24. Silver AL, Lindsay RW, Cheney ML, et al. Thin-profile platinum eyelid weighting: a superior option in the paralyzed eye. Plast Reconstr Surg 2009;123:1697.
25. Chu EA, Byrne PJ. Treatment considerations in facial paralysis. Facial Plast Surg 2008;24:164–9.
26. Henstrom DK, Malo JS, Cheney ML, et al. Platysmectomy: an effective intervention for facial synkinesis and hypertonicity. Arch Facial Plast Surg 2011;13(4):239–43.
27. Sardesai MG, Moe K. Recent progress in facial paralysis: advances and obstacles [review]. Curr Opin Otolaryngol Head Neck Surg 2010;18(4):266–71.
28. Balliet R, Shinn JB, Bach-y-Rita P. Facial paralysis rehabilitation: retraining selective muscle control. Int Rehabil Med 1982;4(2):67–74.
29. Perry ES, Potter NL, Rambo KD, et al. Effects of strength training on neuromuscular facial rehabilitation. Dev Neurorehabil 2011;14(3):164–70.
30. Cronin GW, Steenersion RL. The effectiveness of neuromuscular facial retraining combined with electromyography in facial paralysis rehabilitation. Otolaryngol Head Neck Surg 2003;128:534–8.
31. Manikandan N. Effect of facial neuromuscular re-education on facial symmetry in patients with Bell's palsy: a randomized controlled trial. Clin Rehabil 2007;21(4): 338–43.
32. Ross B, Nedzelski JM, Mclean JA. Efficacy of feedback training in long-standing facial nerve paresis. Laryngoscope 1991;101:744–50.

33. Nakamura K, Toda N, Sakamari K, et al. Biofeedback rehabilitation for the prevention of synkinesis after facial palsy. Otolaryngol Head Neck Surg 2003;128: 539–43.
34. Cardoso JR, Teixeira EC, Moreira MD, et al. Effects of exercises on Bell's palsy; systematic review of randomized controlled trials. Otol Neurotol 2008;29(557): 560.
35. Angelov DN, Ceynowa M, Guntinas-Lichius O, et al. Mechanical stimulation of paralyzed vibrissal muscles following facial nerve injury in adult rat promotes full recovery of whisking. Neurobiol Dis 2007;26(1):229–42.
36. Lal D, Hetzler LT, Sharma N, et al. Electrical stimulation facilitates rat facial nerve recovery from a crush injury. Otolaryngol Head Neck Surg 2008;139(1):68–73.
37. Hadlock T, Lindsay R, Edwards C, et al. The effect of electrical and mechanical stimulation on the regenerating rodent facial nerve. Laryngoscope 2010;120(6): 1094–102.
38. Cai ZG, Shi XJ, Lu XG, et al. Efficacy of functional training of the facial muscles for treatment of incomplete peripheral facial nerve injury. Chin J Dent Res 2010; 13(1):37–43.
39. Greywoode JD, Ho HH, Artz GJ, et al. Management of traumatic facial nerve injuries. Facial Plast Surg 2010;26:511–8.

Reconstruction of the Avulsed Auricle after Trauma

Ralph Magritz, MD*, Ralf Siegert, MD, DDS, PhD

KEYWORDS

- Ear avulsion • Auricular trauma • Ear reattachment • Auricular defect
- Auricular reconstruction

KEY POINTS

- The success of a classic replantation as a composite graft is particularly dependent on the size of the amputated auricle segment and on the associated size and surface of the nutrient base.
- An important criterion for surgery planning is, in addition to localization, the size of the defect, its surface area, and depth.
- Small peripheral defects of the cranial third of the auricle may be reconstructed with typically cranially based transposition flaps.
- Fitting auricular defects, especially subtotal and total defects, with prosthetics plays an important role in the regimen of the reconstructive ear surgeon.

INTRODUCTION

Severe auricular trauma, especially complete amputations, is a rare injury. To date, less than 100 of these have been reported in the literature.

In addition to the type of injury, the location and the extent of the involved auricular structures have an important influence on the selection of an appropriate replantation or reattachment technique. The treatment options vary substantially, ranging from a simple restitching as composite graft up to a complex microvascular replantation.

A satisfactory primary reconstruction is not always possible to obtain and the remaining defects must be reconstructed secondary. The localization of the defect, its extent, and the condition of the tissue surrounding the defect are essential criteria for a further treatment planning.

Disclosure: There is no financial interest or any conflict of interest associated with this work by the authors.

Department of Oto-Rhino-Laryngology, Head and Neck Surgery, Prosper-Hospital, Academic Teaching Hospital, Ruhr University Bochum, Muehlenstrasse 27, Recklinghausen 45659, Germany

* Corresponding author.

E-mail addresses: ralphmagritz@web.de; ralph.magritz@prosper-hospital.de

This article provides an overview of the treatment of acute auricular trauma and important aspects of secondary defect repair of the pinna.

SURGERY OF AURICULAR TRAUMA
Classification

Different classifications of auricular trauma are described in the literature. Some are related to specific causes of injury (eg, sharp or blunt trauma, burn, chemical burn); others consider anatomic landmarks of the ear and the nature and extent of tissue trauma or tissue loss.[1,2] For clinical aspects Weerda's classification into four degrees of injuries[3] has proved to be very useful (**Table 1**).

Superficial Trauma (First Degree)

These cases are characterized by abrasions without or only a little cartilage involvement. The wounds are rinsed and the wound edges adapted and carefully sutured. Small defects are closed with small local skin flaps.

Tear with Nutrient Skin Pedicle (Second Degree)

Primary readaptation of the partially amputated part of the auricle is the best solution in these cases (**Fig. 1**). Because of the excellent vascular supply of the auricle with many branches communicating with each other, even subtotal amputations with a very narrow skin pedicle (6 mm in width) can be reconstructed successfully.[4]

Partial and Total Avulsion with Existing Segment (Third Degree)

The success of a classic replantation as a composite graft is particularly dependent on the size of the amputated auricle segment and on the associated size and surface of the nutrient base. However, the ischemic time of the amputated segment, which usually amounts to less than 4 to 6 hours,[5] can almost be neglected based on animal studies by Weerda and colleagues[6] and does not influence the success or failure of a direct replantation as a composite graft, even in microsurgical replantation.[7,8] Direct reattachment as a composite graft can be achieved when the amputated part is smaller than 15 mm in diameter.[9]

A direct readaptation of larger segments is rarely successful (**Fig. 2**). Therefore, multistaged so-called pocket methods have been suggested. Their common characteristic is that the skin of the amputated auricle is in part or completely removed from the cartilage. The cartilage itself is then stored in a well-vascularized pocket, either

Table 1	
Classification of auricular trauma according to Weerda	
Classification of Auricular Trauma	
First degree	Abrasions without significant cartilage involvement
Second degree	Tear with nutrient skin pedicle
Third degree	Avulsion without segmental loss: Partial avulsion Total avulsion
Fourth degree	Avulsion with segmental loss: Partial defect Total auricular loss

Data from Weerda H. Chirurgie der Ohrmuschel-Verletzungen, Defekte und Anomalien. Stuttgart (Germany): Thieme; 2004.

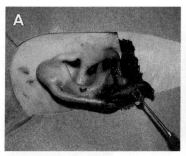
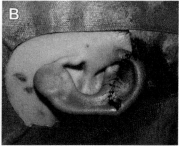

Fig. 1. Pedicled partial amputation of the auricle (second degree). (*A*) Preoperative situation. (*B*) Situation after primary repair.

in the ear region[10,11] or remote area (abdominal,[12,13] supraclavicular,[14] cervical[15,16]). Other authors suggest repositioning of the cartilage and covering it with local skin flaps,[17] with platysma,[18] or with a temporoparietal fascia flap.[19,20]

Another technique to salvage and reconstruct an amputated auricle has been described by Baudet and coworkers.[21] He removes the posterior skin of the amputated auricle; creates little windows into the cartilage in the triangular fossa, scaphoid fold, and cavum conchae to allow an exposure and contact of the underside of the anterior skin to the vascularized bed; and replants it into its original position (**Fig. 3**). He leaves the anterior skin intact and sutured it to the mastoid skin. In a second step some months later the auricle is lifted up and the retroauricular sulcus reconstructed with a skin graft.

The most important problem of all these techniques is a very high failure rate of about 60%.[3] In addition, the delicate elastic cartilage is unable to withstand the contractile forces of scarring especially when using the pocket principle including its modifications. Because of distortion and flattening the contours of the auricular cartilage are lost in time so that the esthetic results are not convincing in a high number of cases.

In 1980, Pennington and colleagues[22] reported the first successful microsurgical replantation of an auricle using vein grafts to the superficial artery and vein. Compared

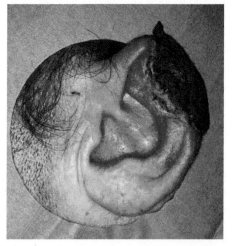

Fig. 2. Necrosis of a medium-sized replant after a classic replantation.

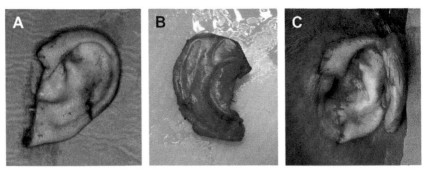

Fig. 3. Replantation using Baudet's technique. (*A*) Avulsed auricle segment. (*B*) Situation after removal of the posterior skin and fenestration of the cartilage. (*C*) Reattached auricle.

with all other techniques microsurgical replantation offers the best chance for success and shows excellent aesthetic results. Nevertheless, microvascular replantation is very challenging, not only because of the small vessel diameter less than 1 mm.[23] Depending on the type of injury, an additional vessel damage by stretching and pressure may occur with an increasing risk of vascular complications, especially on venous congestion.[24] A suitable vein cannot always be found in the amputated part, sometimes not even after successful arterial revascularization.[25] In such cases and in cases of visible venous congestion it is essential to prevent or reduce a venous backflow problem using multiple skin punctures, stitch incisions, and leeches.[26] Regarding several reports that venous connections between the replanted auricle and the recipient bed occur within a week after replantation, a venous drainage procedure should be performed during that time period.[27–30]

The technique by Baudet can be summarized as an appropriate second choice if a microsurgical replantation is not possible.[21,31,32] However, the pocket techniques should no longer be used.

Partial and Total Avulsion without Existing Segment (Fourth Degree)

Severe injuries to the auricular region with loss of the amputated auricle or auricle segment have to be covered by local skin flaps or free skin grafts. After some months the auricle can then be reconstructed secondary.

SECONDARY RECONSTRUCTION OF AURICULAR DEFECTS

Defects and deformities of the auricle are not only caused by accidents or trauma. In addition they are the result of tumor resections and rarely of complications of aesthetic or reconstructive surgery using improper techniques. The techniques of reconstruction are, with the exception of the correction of microtia, in essence identical and follow standardized surgical principles.[33]

Classification

An important criterion for surgery planning is, in addition to localization, the size of the defect and its surface area and depth. Based on the aforementioned variables, auricular defects may be classified simply and reproducibly in the everyday clinical setting (**Table 2**).

Moreover, the integrity of the tissue surrounding the defect is very important. Scar tissue, previous surgery, and previous radiation therapy may greatly affect and limit

Table 2 Classification of auricular defects according to Weerda and Siegert		
Classification of Auricular Defects		
Central	**Peripheral**	**Postauricular**
Ear channel	Helix	
Concha	Upper part	**Subtotal**
Antihelix	Medial part	
Combined	Lower part, lobule	**Total**

Data from Weerda H, Siegert R. Classification and treatment of acquired deformities. Face 1998;6:79–82.

the techniques used. Therefore, this must be taken into consideration for surgery planning.

Central Defects

Skin defects of the concha are most effectively treated with a full-thickness skin graft as long as the perichondrium is intact. If not, the cartilage should be removed and a skin graft sutured onto the vascularized connective tissue underneath the cartilage. The retroauricular region of the ipsilateral, or alternatively, the contralateral side serves as the donor area.

Multilayer defects of the concha and the adjacent antihelix may be reconstructed with a cranial- or caudal-based retroauricular pedicled flap. Its pedicle can be severed after 2 to 3 weeks. This procedure may be performed in a similar manner to a transposition flap with a portion of pedicle epithelium being removed for tunneling or with a subcutaneous pedicled island flap from the postauricular sulcus.

The pedicle containing the posterior auricularis artery may be placed cranially or caudally. This is possible because of the perfusion in the case of a cranially based flap.

In extended central defects including the antihelix a large retroauricular cranially based bilobed flap by Weerda[3] may be used. The antihelix should be reconstructed with rib cartilage (**Fig. 4**).

Because of visible scaring, the use of preauricular flaps should be the exception. In such cases a cranial pedicle should be used to align the scar strictly in the preauricular fold.

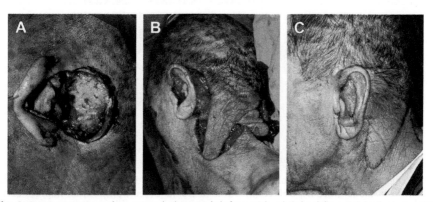

Fig. 4. Reconstruction of an extended central defect with a bilobed flap. (*A*) Defect size. (*B*) Flap design. (*C*) Result after some months.

Peripheral Defects

Small peripheral defects of the cranial third of the auricle may be reconstructed with typically cranially based transposition flaps. For the reconstruction of the helix cartilage, it is advisable to use a concha cartilage transplant, optimally from the ipsilateral side. The pedicle may be severed about 3 weeks after the operation and replaced in the retroauricular donor region. To obtain a harmonic continuity of the helix, the flap should be carefully melded into the defect area (**Fig. 5**).

A further most suitable method of reconstructing small defects of the cranial third of the auricle is Gersuny's technique[34] as modified by Anita and Buch.[35] Although it is a so-called reduction technique, this method leads to a negligible reduction in the craniocaudal size of the auricle and can be performed as a one-step procedure. The chondrocutaneous sliding flaps should be prepared in a two-layered manner while protecting the posterior skin (**Fig. 6**).

In cases of larger defects with loss of the upper third of the auricle, we prefer a multi-step procedure using costal cartilage. The first operative step involves reconstruction of the cartilage defect with costal cartilage. The costal cartilage is carved using a template made from the contralateral ear. Typically, we use the cartilaginous portion of the seventh rib. The cartilaginous framework should be approximately 3 mm smaller in all dimensions than the template (ie, than the defect itself). After preparation of a skin pocket whose incision lies cranially of the defect and into the hairy portion of the scalp, the framework is attached to the auricular cartilage using several slowly absorbable sutures. Through application of a suction drain, the thinly prepared skin adheres to

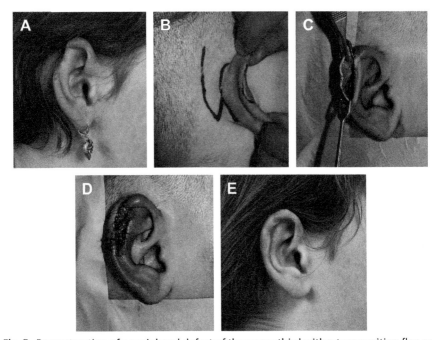

Fig. 5. Reconstruction of a peripheral defect of the upper third with a transposition flap and a concha cartilage graft. (*A*) Defect. (*B*) Outlined cranial based transposition flap. (*C*) Cartilage graft. (*D*) Situation at the end of the first step. (*E*) Situation several months after severing the pedicle.

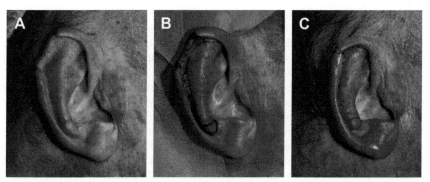

Fig. 6. Reconstruction of a peripheral defect using Gersuny's technique. (A) Defect. (B) Outlined resection of skin and underlying cartilage. (C) Result at the end of the operation.

the cartilage template like wallpaper. Here it is especially important to have an optimal fit between the framework of the rib cartilage and the remaining auricular cartilage. These two components should be tapered and positioned such that there are no palpable edges (**Fig. 7**).

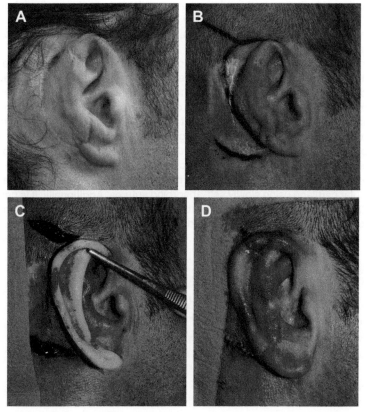

Fig. 7. Reconstruction of a larger peripheral defect using rib cartilage. (A) Defect. (B) Outlined skin incisions (oblique). (C) Carved partial auricular framework using the seventh rib. (D) Situation at the end of the operation.

During a second surgical step around 6 months later the auricle is detached from the undersurface together with its surrounding connective tissue and the retroauricular crease is formed. The elevated position of the auricle is stabilized with an additional piece of rib cartilage, which is covered with a fascia flap either of the superficial temporal fascia or mastoid fascia. The remaining defect is covered with a skin graft.

Common techniques for the reconstruction of small peripheral defects of the middle third of the auricle are the so-called wedge excisions with their many variants.[3] However, to obtain an aesthetically pleasing result, a certain amount of skill and intuition in the planning stage and in the excision typically of several Burow triangles is necessary.

A more elegant and aesthetically pleasing result for middle third auricular defects is obtained using a modified Gersuny technique and thus is the method we favor to the wedge excision. Both the wedge excision and the modified Gerunsy technique lead to a decrease in auricle size. This must be discussed with the patient before surgery.

Should this decrease in auricle size be too severe or should the patient deny the procedure, a two-step retroauricular transposition flap similar to that used in defects of the cranial third of the auricle may be used for the reconstruction of small to mid-sized helical defects of the middle auricular third.

Along the same line of reconstruction without a decrease in auricular size, large defects of the middle auricular third may be reconstructed using a single-step retroauricular Burow's sliding or U-flap. The cartilaginous helix is reconstructed using the aforementioned technique with ipsilateral or contralateral concha cartilage transplantation. Extensive peripheral defects of the middle third of the auricle, most often in combination with central auricular defects, require a multistep reconstruction using costal cartilage.

Circumscript defects of the caudal third of the auricle including the lobe are reconstructed in two steps typically using either cranial- or caudal-based retroauricular pedicled flaps. The surgical procedure is comparable with the previously mentioned auricular reconstruction techniques for the cranial and medial defects. Only in exceptions should the surgeon forego the use of cartilage from concha or rib to obtain an aesthetically pleasing, stable, and enduring result.

Complete loss of the ear lobe is reconstructed in one step using a Gavello pedicled transposition flap.[1] To preserve a harmonic lobe contour, a stable support of concha or rib cartilage ought to be embedded into the lobe and attached to the caudal end of the auricular cartilage using slowly self-absorbing sutures. Additionally, it is necessary to plan the flap such that the anterior portion is slightly larger than the posterior. This allows for an aesthetically well-positioned retroauricular scar (**Fig. 8**).

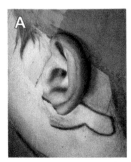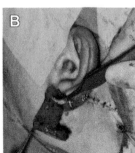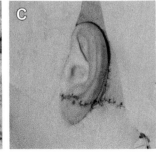

Fig. 8. Reconstruction of a lobule defect using a ventral-based Gavello flap and a concha cartilage graft. (*A*) Defect and outlined flap design. (*B*) Elevated flap and support with a concha cartilage graft. (*C*) Result at the end of the operation.

Extensive lower auricular third defects including the lobe are reconstructed using a stabile partial costal cartilage frame in conjunction with retroauricular and infra-auricular advancement flaps (**Fig. 9**). If it is not feasible to form the retroauricular sulcus simultaneously, then a second step should be performed in which the reconstructed lower third of the auricle is detached and covered laterally (retroauricularly) and medially with skin grafts.

Subtotal and Total Defects

The reconstruction of subtotal and complete auricle loss is a true surgical challenge. The state of the tissue and scar tissue surrounding the remaining auricle and the remaining auricle itself is of particular significance. The success of auricular reconstruction is negatively correlated to the amount of scar tissue in the defect area.

Should there be only mild scarring in the defect area and should the scar tissue be centrally located at the same level as the concha, then one can expect a good outcome of a multistep reconstruction using local skin and a costal cartilage framework.

In the case of extensive scarring, it is possible to increase the area of unscarred tissue using a tissue expander under the intact skin (**Fig. 10**). The expander is filled with normal saline solution 2 weeks after implantation with additional fluid being added for 8 to 12 weeks. The explantation of the expander takes place simultaneously with the implantation of the costal cartilage framework in an orthotopic position under the expanded tissue. The connective tissue capsule that has formed around the expander should be removed before implantation. Using a suction drain for 4 to 5 days postoperatively, we are able to do without the use of sutures for cartilage fixation. In a second operation, the auricle is elevated and the retroauricular sulcus constructed as described previously.

In principle, the use of a temporoparietal fascia flap pedicled on the posterior branch of the superficial temporal artery is a single-step alternative to the aforementioned expander method in cases of extensive scarring at the site of reconstruction. Such a fascia flap, if large enough, can completely cover an cartilage framework of the auricle and, as opposed to the multistep methods, provides an a priori retroauricular support. The fascia flap is then covered with a split-skin graft (0.3 mm) from the scalp (**Fig. 11**).

If the fascia is present but the vascular supply of the temporoparietal fascia flap by the superficial temporal vessels inadequate because of scarring or previous surgery, then it is advisable to form a wide pedicle as in a random pattern flap. In this case, the flap receives its blood supply from the posterior auricular and occipital vessels, which taken alone would mean a somewhat less dependable perfusion. However, using a

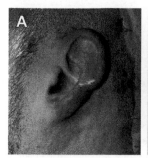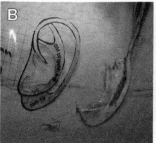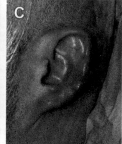

Fig. 9. Reconstruction of an extended defect of the lower third. (*A*) Defect. (*B*) Carved partial auricular framework using the seventh rib. (*C*) Situation at the end of the operation.

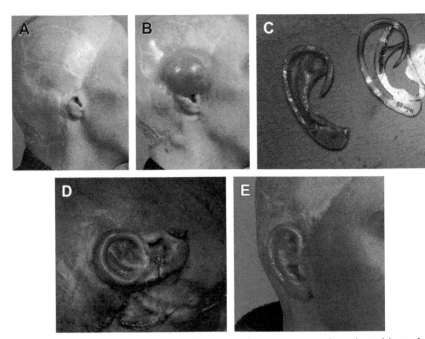

Fig. 10. Reconstruction of the auricle after an avulsion trauma and a subtotal loss of the auricle. (*A*) Defect. (*B*) Situation 3 months after skin expander implantation. (*C*) Carved and sculptured auricular framework. (*D*) Situation after skin expander removal and implantation of the auricular framework. (*E*) Final result several months after elevation of the auricle within a second surgical step.

wide pedicle containing occipital and other temporal collaterals is reliable and recommended. Such a reconstruction should be performed in two steps (**Fig. 12**).

Should the temporoparietal fascia no longer be available and should the scar tissue be so extensive that skin expansion seems unfeasible, then a microvascularly

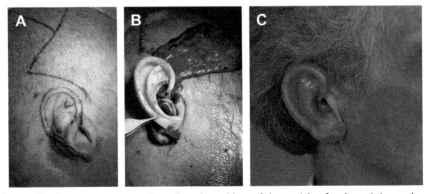

Fig. 11. Single-stage reconstruction of a subtotal loss of the auricle after burn injury using a pedicled temporoparietal fascia flap (TPF-flap), rib cartilage, and a split-skin graft from the scalp. (*A*) Defect, outlined position of the auricle, and marked incisions for TPF-flap elevation. (*B*) Auricular framework and elevated TPF-flap. (*C*) Final result 1 year postoperative.

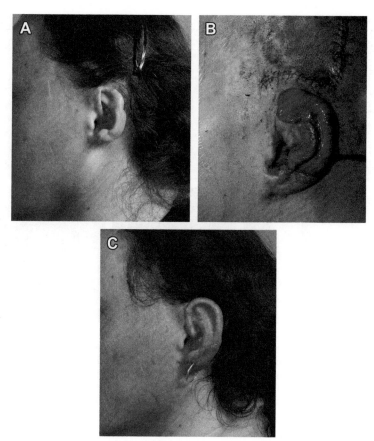

Fig. 12. Staged reconstruction of a subtotal amputated auricle using a wide pedicled TPF-flap, rib cartilage, and split-skin grafts from the head. (*A*) Defect. (*B*) Situation right after implantation of the auricular framework and covering with a wide TPF-flap (note the extended scarring in the frontotemporal area right above the superficial temporal vessels). (*C*) Final result 1 year after elevation of the auricle and reconstruction of the retroauricular sulcus within a second surgical step.

reanastomized contralateral free fascia flap may be used. The graft should be connected to the superficial temporal or facial vessels. An alternative to the temporoparietal free fascia flap is the free forearm fascia flap with microvascular revascularization, as described previously. The operation can take place in a single step.

Under the same circumstances, the preparation of a prelaminated forearm flap with a cartilaginous auricle framework is also possible (**Fig. 13**). The surgery becomes a two-step procedure. In the first step, the rib cartilage is harvested and the auricular framework formed. The framework is then implanted between the radial forearm fascia and the finely dissected forearm skin. The second step takes place 6 months later at which point the preformed forearm flap is harvested, brought into orthotopic position and microsurgically revascularized. In principle, during this step the retroauricular sulcus may be formed using a costal cartilage wedge, local pedicled flaps, and split-skin grafts from the scalp, thus making an additional step unnecessary.

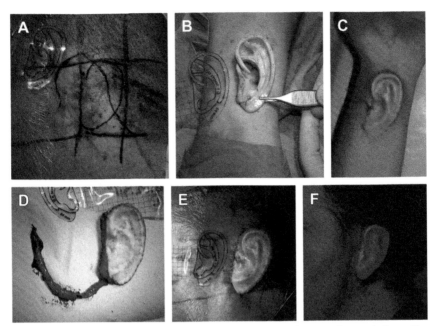

Fig. 13. Auricular reconstruction using a prelaminated radial forearm flap and rib cartilage. (A) Extended scarring after several previous operations for bone-anchored prosthesis in a microtia patient (marked position of the new auricle and outlined hairline). (B) Auricular framework right before implantation in the left forearm. (C) Situation 6 months later. (D) Harvested prelaminated forearm flap including its pedicle. (E) Situation after positioning of the auricle and microvascular flap revascularization. (F) Result 6 months postoperative.

Prosthetic Rehabilitation

Fitting auricular defects, especially subtotal and total defects, with prosthetics plays an important role in the regimen of the reconstructive ear surgeon. Prosthetics are indicated whenever the requirements for the typically multistep surgical reconstruction are not met, when the general health of the patient does not allow for surgery, and always when the patient does not wish to have an auricular reconstruction.

Prosthetics may be attached in various manners, the easiest being adhesive affixation. This is typically chosen as an interim solution until an auricular reconstruction can take place. Because adhesives are relatively unreliable, they are not viewed as a permanent option for prosthesis anchoring. Additionally, adhesives can cause various degrees of local skin irritation, which can inhibit wearing the prosthesis.

The most widespread technique for prosthesis affixation is by bone-anchored implants. As opposed to adhesives, bone-anchored implants offer an exceptionally secure and stabile mount for a prosthesis. However, the method is not without shortcomings because the patient must clean and care for the percutaneous implant sites daily. Despite this, recurring infection and formation of granulation around the implant sites are not uncommon. A loosening of the implants or even implant loss is rare.

An alternative to the percutaneous implant is a transcutaneous magnetically coupled prosthesis. The prosthesis is fixed magnetically by a titanium-encapsuled permanent double magnet that has been placed in preformed recesses ground into the petrosal bone and fastened securely with mini osteosynthesis screws. The skin

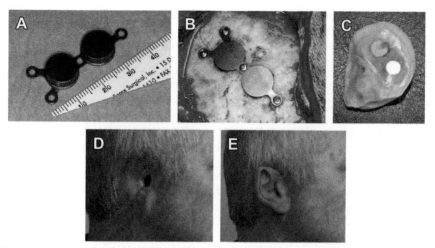

Fig. 14. Transcutaneous prosthetic fixation using implantable double magnets without open implants. (*A*) Implantable double magnets. (*B*) Implant fixed into the temporal bone by screws. (*C*) Prosthesis with incorporated magnets. (*D*) Patient after resection of right auricle because of a carcinoma several years before and after implantation of double magnets. (*E*) Situation when wearing his magnetically fixed prosthesis.

above the magnets remains intact. The prosthesis is then designed with two magnets. The result is a stabile mount that ensures secure attachment of the prosthesis without the shortcomings of an open implant (**Fig. 14**).

REFERENCES

1. Rettinger G, Reichensperger-Goertzen C. Gesichtsverletzungen durch Hundebiß. HNO 1995;3:159–64.
2. Punjabi AP, Haug RH, Jordan RB. Management of injuries to the auricle. J Oral Maxillofac Surg 1997;55:732–9.
3. Weerda H. Chirurgie der Ohrmuschel – Verletzungen, Defekte und Anomalien. Stuttgart: Thieme; 2004.
4. Özelik D, Ünveren T, Toplu G. Subtotal ear amputation with a very narrow pedicle: a case report and review of the literature. Ulus Travma Acil Cerrahi Derg 2009; 15(3):306–10.
5. Pollock FE Jr, Smith TL, Koman LA, Holden MB, Smith BP. Decreased microvascular perfusion in the rabbit ear after six hours of ischemia. J Orthop Res 1994;12: 48–57.
6. Weerda H, Grüner R, Cannive B. Die Einheilungsrate frei transplantierter, großer "Composite grafts". Arch Otorhinolaryngol 1986;(Suppl II):129.
7. Shelley OP, Villafane O, Watson SB. Successful partial ear replantation after prolonged ischemia time. Br J Plast Surg 1999;53:76e7.
8. Wong W, Wilson P, Savundra J. Total ear replantation using the distal radial artery perforator. J Plast Reconstr Aesthet Surg 2011;64(5):677–9.
9. Ihrai T, Balaguer T, Monteil MC, Chignon-Sicard B, Médard de Chardon V, Riah Y, Lebreton E. Surgical management of traumatic ear amputations: literature review. Ann Chir Plast Esthet 2009;54(2):146–51.
10. Mladick R, Horton C, Adamson J, Cohen B. The pocket principle. Plast Reconstr Surg 1971;48:219–23.

11. Mladick R, Carraway J. Ear reattachement by the modified pocket principle. Plast Reconstr Surg 1973;51:584–7.

12. Conway H, Neumann CG, Gelb J, Leveridge LL, Joseph JM. Reconstruction of the external ear. Ann Surg 1948;128:226–38.

13. Musgrave RH, Garrett WS. Management of avulsion injuries of the external ear. Plast Reconstr Surg 1967;40:534–9.

14. Spira M. Early care of deformities of the auricle resulting from mechanical trauma. In: Tanzer RC, Edgerton MT, editors. Symposium on reconstruction of the auricle. St Louis (MO): CV Mosby & Co; 1974. p. 204–17, X.

15. Conroy W. Letter to the editor: Salvage of an amputated ear. Plast Reconstr Surg 1972;49:564.

16. de Mello-Filho FV, Mamede RCM, Koury AP. Use of a platysma myocutaneous flap for the reimplantation of a severed ear: Experience with five cases. Sao Paulo Med J 1999;117:218–23.

17. Elsahy N. Ear replantation combined with local flaps. Ann Plast Surg 1986;77: 102–11.

18. Ariyan S, Chicarilli Z. Replantation of a totally amputated ear by means of a platysma musculocutaneous "sandwich" flap. Plast Reconstr Surg 1986;78: 385–9.

19. Jenkins AM, Finucan T. Primary nonmicrosurgical reconstruction following ear avulsion using the temporoparietal fascial island flap. Plast Reconstr Surg 1989;83(1):148–52.

20. Saad Ibrahim SM, Zidan A, Madani S. Totally avulsed ear: new technique of immediate ear reconstruction. J Plast Reconstr Aesthet Surg 2008;61(Suppl 1): S29–36.

21. Baudet J, Tramond P, Gonmain A. A propos d'un procede original de reimplantation d'un pavillon de l'oreille totalement separe. Ann Chir Plast Esthet 1972;17: 67–72.

22. Pennington DG, Lai MF, Pelly AD. Successful replantation of a completely avulsed ear by microvascular anastomosis. Plast Reconstr Surg 1980;65:820–3.

23. Shen XQ, Wang C, Xu JH, Wu SC. Successful microsurgical replantation of a child's completely amputated ear. J Plast Reconstr Aesthet Surg 2008;61(12): e19–22.

24. Kind GM, Buncke GM, Placik OJ, et al. Total ear replantation. Plast Reconstr Surg 1997;99:1858–67.

25. Concannon MJ, Puckett CL. Microsurgical replantation of an ear in a child without venous repair. Plast Reconstr Surg 1998;102:2088–93.

26. Akyürek M, Safak T, Keçik A. Microsurgical ear replantation without venous repair: failure of development of venous channels despite patency of arterial anastomosis for 14 days. Ann Plast Surg 2001;46(4):439–42.

27. Cho BH, Ahn HB. Microsurgical replantation of a partial ear with leech therapy. Ann Plast Surg 1999;43:427–9.

28. de Chalain T, Jones G. Replantation of the avulsed pinna: 100 percent survival with a single arterial anastomosis and substitution of leeches for a venous anastomosis. Plast Reconstr Surg 1995;95:1275–9.

29. Safak T, Özcan G, Keçik A, et al. Microvascular ear replantation with no vein anastomosis. Plast Reconstr Surg 1993;92:945–8.

30. Juri J, Irigary A, Juri C, Grilli D, Blanco CM, Vasquez GD. Ear replantation. Plast Reconstr Surg 1987;80:431–4.

31. Horta R, Costa-Ferreira A, Costa J, Silva P, Amarante JM, Silva A, Filipe R. Ear replantation after human bite avulsion injury. J Craniofac Surg 2011;22(4):1457–9.

32. Kyrmizakis DE, Karatzanis AD, Bourolias CA, Hadjiioannou JK, Velegrakis GA. Nonmicrosurgical reconstruction of the auricle after traumatic amputation due to human bite. Head Face Med 2006;2:45.
33. Siegert R, Magritz R. Reconstruction of the auricle. GMS Curr Top Otorhinolaryngol Head Neck Surg 2007;6:Doc02. Epub 2008 Mar 14.
34. Gersuny R. Über einige kosmetische Operationen. Wien Med Wschr 1903;48: 2253–7.
35. Anita N, Buch V. Chondrocutaneous advancement flap for the marginal defects of the ear. Plast Reconstr Surg 1967;39:472–7.

Secondary Repair of Acquired Enophthalmos

Joseph N. Giacometti, MD[a],*, Seongmu Lee, MD[b],
Michael T. Yen, MD[a]

KEYWORDS

- Orbital trauma • Enophthalmos • Orbital fracture • Orbital surgery
- Secondary repair • Enophthalmic wedge implant

KEY POINTS

- Enophthalmos is a potential sequela in trauma patients with orbital fractures; when necessary, primary surgical repair of the orbital fractures should be performed soon after the initial injury.
- Occasionally, patients present with persistent clinically significant enophthalmos after primary surgical repair.
- The therapeutic approach of persistent clinically significant enophthalmos after primary repair depends on the degree of orbital and facial asymmetry and the presence of residual soft tissue incarceration.
- Enophthalmic wedge implants are an effective and safe option for patients with persistent postoperative enophthalmos who require secondary surgical repair.

POSTTRAUMATIC ENOPHTHALMOS

Enophthalmos, defined as the recession of the globe within the bony orbital compartment, is a common sequela of facial trauma involving orbital fractures. The condition develops secondary to displacement of a constant volume of orbital soft tissue in the setting of mechanical disruption and expansion of the bony structure of the orbit.[1,2] Orbital fractures allow shifting of the orbital tissues into the adjacent sinuses. Fractures of the medial and inferior walls, the most common orbital fracture sites, lead to orbital fat prolapse into the ethmoid and maxillary sinuses, respectively.[3–5] This

Funding sources: No outside funding was received for this article.
Conflict of interest: Nil (J.N. Giacometti, S. Lee); Consultant for Merz Pharmaceuticals (Frankfurt, Germany) (M.T. Yen).
[a] Department of Ophthalmology, Cullen Eye Institute, Baylor College of Medicine, 1977 Butler Boulevard, Houston, TX 77030, USA; [b] Private Practice, 14445 Olive View Drive, Sylmar, Los Angeles, CA 91342, USA
* Corresponding author.
E-mail address: giacomet@bcm.edu

Otolaryngol Clin N Am 46 (2013) 857–866
http://dx.doi.org/10.1016/j.otc.2013.06.005
0030-6665/13/$ – see front matter © 2013 Elsevier Inc. All rights reserved.

posttraumatic migration of orbital soft tissue results in the globe shifting to a more posterior, and frequently more inferior, position. In their retrospective review of 119 cases of unilateral orbital fractures, He and colleagues[6] found that combined medial-inferior wall fractures were responsible for most cases of posttraumatic enophthalmos.

Small amounts of enophthalmos (less than 3 mm) are undetectable and clinically insignificant.[7,8] However, when patients sustain severe trauma involving larger fractures of the orbital walls, the resulting enophthalmos (3 mm or greater) can be quite obvious and aesthetically unacceptable (**Fig. 1**). Furthermore, because the extraocular muscles are frequently also displaced by the shifting of orbital tissues, diplopia may occur.[2,9] Surgical repair of the associated fractures is necessary in these instances to restore both structure and function.

Traditionally, autologous tissue implants were used for orbital reconstruction, including grafts from iliac, mandibular, maxillary, rib, and calvarial bone.[10–12] More recently, the options for donor graft site have expanded to include more accessible tissue, such as nasal septum and anterior maxillary sinus wall.[13,14] Although the autologous option offers seamless integration of the grafts into host tissue with low rates of extrusion, it also requires longer operating time and is associated with donor site morbidity.[15] Over the past several years, there have been significant advancements in the manufacture of highly biocompatible alloplastic orbital implants. Surgeons now have many options when choosing an alloplastic implant, including resorbable and nonresorbable materials.[16–21] Resorbable implants have the advantage of minimal inflammatory response and scarring at the expense of a decline in tensile strength over time (ie, polydioxanone). Nonresorbable implants have become very popular recently and include high-density porous polyethylene and titanium. These implants allow for integration of native tissue and offer good long-term stability. However, the presence of a permanent foreign body in the orbit confers a low risk of implant migration, exposure, extrusion, or infection. When surgeons choose implants appropriately and use sound surgical technique, orbital fracture repair has a very good success rate with regard to the correction of posttraumatic enophthalmos and the complication rates are low.

PERSISTENT ENOPHTHALMOS AFTER PRIMARY ORBITAL FRACTURE REPAIR
Nature of the Problem and Indications for Secondary Repair

In up to 10% of cases after primary repair of orbital fractures, patients present with persistent postoperative enophthalmos despite a seemingly successful reconstruction of the bony defect.[22] This deformity may or may not be apparent in the immediate postoperative period. In some instances, enophthalmos may develop slowly over

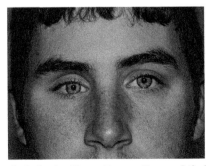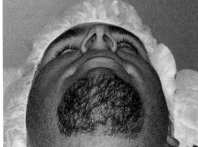

Fig. 1. Patient with posttraumatic enophthalmos and hypoglobus of the right eye.

several months as postoperative edema resolves. Over this time, surrounding periorbital tissues heal, remodel, and may contract, and the orbital fat may also atrophy.

Factors that may be associated with persistent enophthalmos after primary fracture repair include a severe initial bony deformity, excessively delayed initial surgery, or inadequate initial repair.[23] In particular, the timing of the primary repair has significant importance. Surgeons should aim to perform the primary repair soon after the traumatic event. Although most surgeons prefer to wait for some resolution in the normal posttraumatic edema, over a 1-year period following initial injury, several irreversible soft tissue changes take place within the orbit. These alterations may subsequently lead to permanent deformities in the underlying skeletal structure, and ultimately make repair extremely difficult.[24] Imola and colleagues[23] found that primary repair should ideally be performed at least within 3 to 6 months after acute injury for the best possibility of attaining restoration of facial form.

Indications for secondary repair of acquired clinically significant enophthalmos are similar to those for primary repair. Specifically, when enophthalmos is significant enough to cause aesthetically unacceptable facial asymmetry or when the deformity is accompanied by periorbital soft-tissue incarceration with functional compromise (ie, extraocular motility restriction and/or diplopia), secondary correction should be pursued. In terms of the timing of secondary repair, it is important to wait for resolution of postoperative edema after the primary repair to appreciate the true amount of residual enophthalmos.

Secondary Enophthalmos Repair: Management Options

Options for secondary repair of enophthalmos can generally be broken down into 2 broad categories: surgical and minimally invasive. Surgical correction involves orbital exploration and liberation of any residual soft tissue incarceration along with mechanical repositioning of the orbital contents via secondary implant placement. The minimally invasive option includes periocular injection of alloplastic materials with the goal of orbital volume augmentation.

For patients who require surgical management, surgeons may use any of the many autologous or alloplastic implants previously mentioned in this article. The authors' preference for most cases of secondary clinically significant enophthalmos repair is to use the high-density porous polyethylene wedge implant. Similar to other high-density porous polyethylene implants, wedge implants have the advantage of good fibrovascular tissue integration. In addition, the "wedge" shape provides the bulk of volume augmentation posteriorly behind the globe with a thicker midsection and tapered anterior and posterior edges (**Fig. 2**). When the thicker central portion is appropriately positioned inferior and posterior to the globe, it adds volume and exerts an anterosuperior force that helps correct both enophthalmos and hypoglobus.[25] Traditionally, wedge implants have been used in anophthalmic patients with sunken socket syndrome for orbital volume augmentation. Recent studies have also shown them to be effective and safe in the primary correction of posttraumatic enophthalmos in seeing eyes.[25,26] In the authors' experience, enophthalmic wedge implants are very useful in secondary repairs as well.

Periocular injection of various biocompatible materials is an alternative, minimally invasive option for the secondary repair of clinically significant enophthalmos. The most popular injectable modalities include hydrophilic hydrogel pellet tissue self-expanders (**Fig. 3**) and dermal filler injections, such as calcium hydroxylapatite spheres and hyaluronic acid.[27–32] Although most published studies have investigated these materials as volume-enhancing treatments of anophthalmic sockets with

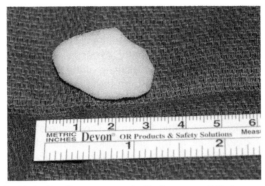

Fig. 2. Top view of a high-density porous polyethylene enophthalmos wedge implant.

enophthalmos and/or socket contracture, their utility can also be extrapolated to the secondary correction of posttraumatic enophthalmos in seeing eyes.

Decision-making: Surgical Versus Minimally-invasive Management

To determine the ideal method of correcting residual enophthalmos for each patient, surgeons should obtain a thorough history and physical examination. If possible, complete records describing the primary repair should be obtained, including preoperative imaging, operative reports, and information on the type and size of implant or graft used during the primary repair.

With regard to presenting symptoms, if a patient is complaining of persistent diplopia with accompanying abnormalities in extraocular motility, it is possible there is some residual incarceration of orbital soft tissue. Therefore, surgical exploration and repair will likely be necessary. Preoperative evaluation with orbital imaging should be undertaken in these circumstances to determine the location and the amount of involved soft tissue. Occasionally, imaging may reveal a poorly positioned primary implant that is impinging on an extraocular muscle; this would also be an indication for surgical correction.

Some patients may have no symptoms other than noticing an asymmetric facial appearance. In this situation, if extraocular motility is full with no evidence of periorbital soft tissue entrapment, the therapeutic decision-making should then depend on the relative amount of enophthalmos present. This amount of enophthalmos can be best measured using Hertel's exophthalmometry. Small amounts of asymmetry (less than 3 mm) should be amenable to treatment with injectables. Patients with

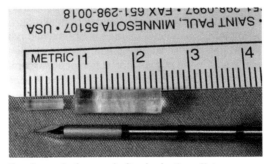

Fig. 3. Hydrogel pellet shown before and after hydration. Sixteen-gauge needle shown for size comparison.

enophthalmos 3 mm or greater or accompanied by significant amounts of hypoglobus will likely need surgical intervention with orbital implant volume augmentation.

For patients meeting criteria for surgical repair, the authors prefer the placement of a high-density porous polyethylene enophthalmic wedge implant. In the next section, the implementation of this surgical modality is discribed.

POROUS POLYETHYLENE ENOPHTHALMIC WEDGE IMPLANT
Preoperative Planning

As discussed in the previous section, imaging of the involved anatomy should be thoroughly reviewed before surgery to assess positioning of the primary implant and to localize accurately any residual soft tissue or bony abnormalities (**Fig. 4**). This imaging will aid in determining the best surgical approach. Visualizing the extent of pathologic abnormality present can also give the surgeon an estimate as to what size implant might be needed for repair. In general, it is a good idea to have multiple sizes of implants available, including one size smaller and one size larger than your estimate. It is important to make sure before the procedure that appropriately sized implants will be available in the operating room on the day of surgery.

Typically the authors perform this procedure in an outpatient ambulatory surgical setting with general anesthesia. Endotracheal intubation is usually preferred because surgical bleeding can flow into the sinuses and posterior pharyngeal space. Patients need to be in good cardiovascular health, and preoperative cardiovascular evaluation and clearance should be obtained when necessary. To reduce the possibility of complications related to excessive intraoperative and postoperative bleeding, patients should temporarily stop all anticoagulants (at least 7 to 10 days for salicylic acid or clopidogrel; at least 3 to 5 days for warfarin), which is frequently coordinated with the patient's primary care provider or cardiologist.

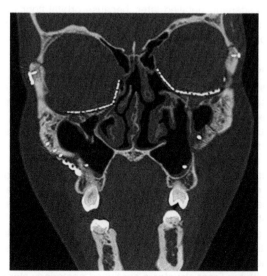

Fig. 4. Computed tomographic image of a patient who presented with clinically significant posttraumatic enophthalmos and hypoglobus. Patient had a history of facial trauma with subsequent repair of multiple fractures, including an orbital floor fracture with a titanium implant on the right side. Note the amount of volume expansion present in the right orbit and the asymmetrical globe position compared with the left.

Patient Preparation and Positioning

In the preoperative area, on establishment of intravenous access, the patient is administered a dose of antibiotics: cefazolin (Ancef; SmithKline Beecham, Philadelphia, PA, USA) or clindamycin (Cleocin; Pfizer, New York, NY, USA). Once in the operating room, the patient is placed in the supine position. The authors prefer a small amount of reverse Trendelenberg position for slight caudal diversion of blood flow to reduce excessive intraoperative bleeding. Continuous cardiac monitoring by an anesthesiologist is essential as intraoperative manipulation of extraocular muscles can induce a vagal response with bradycardia. Once general anesthesia has been induced and the patient's airway secured, administration of local anesthesia can proceed. Lidocaine 2% (with epinephrine 1:100,000) is infiltrated into the inferior conjunctival fornix and lateral canthal region on the operative side. A regional block of the infraorbital nerve may also be given. Lubricant ointment is placed in the nonoperative eye. The patient's entire face is prepped and draped in the usual sterile fashion for orbital surgery.

Procedural Approach

The general surgical principles for placement of a wedge implant are as follows:

- Incision with dissection down to the level of the orbital rim and entrance into orbit.
- Identification of previously placed implant and dissection of any periorbital tissue away from the implant and associated orbital fracture (including scar tissue and extraocular muscle).
- Placement of wedge implant over the original implant.
- Evaluation with forced ductions to check for globe restriction and measurement of amount of residual enophthalmos and/or hypoglobus.
- Closure of incisions.

For the surgical scenario detailed later, because orbital floor fractures are those most commonly associated with enophthalmos, it is assumed that the patient is presenting with enophthalmos after primary floor fracture repair with implant.

Surgical Technique

- Stevens scissors are used to perform a lateral canthotomy and inferior cantholysis; a transconjunctival incision is created in the inferior fornix and extended from the lateral canthal region medially to the caruncle.
- A 4-0 silk suture is placed through the conjunctiva and lower eyelid retractor complex and these tissues are elevated superiorly; the suture is secured with a hemostat.
- Blunt dissection is performed down to the level of the inferior orbital rim (fibrotic scar tissue may be encountered during this and should be dissected away bluntly); once the inferior orbital rim has been reached, the overlying periosteum is incised with a Bard-Parker no. 15 blade.
- A Freer elevator is used to elevate the periorbita off the inferior orbital rim and anterior portion of the orbital floor; the anterior portion of the titanium plate is identified and loose screws should be removed.
- Dissection with the Freer elevator is continued posteriorly along the orbital floor; the orbital tissues are slowly and meticulously dissected away from the titanium implant and dissection is also performed medially and laterally until the entire orbital floor is exposed and adequate space is created for secondary orbital implant placement.

- An enophthalmos wedge implant of predetermined size is placed into the orbit on top of the titanium plate; some carving of the implant can be performed with a blade or surgical scissors.
- The conjunctiva overlying the medial and lateral recti is grasped with toothed forceps and forced duction testing is performed to check for residual restriction; if there is any residual restriction present, additional orbital dissection is performed or the orbital implant size is reduced until the globe moves freely.
- Globe position is assessed to ensure enophthalmos (and hypoglobus) has been adequately corrected; if necessary, the previously placed wedge implant is replaced with a smaller or larger implant. Once adequate globe position is achieved, a titanium screw may be used to fixate the implant to the lateral orbital floor.
- The periosteum along the inferior orbital rim is closed with interrupted 4-0 Polyglactin sutures; the conjunctival fornix incision is closed with interrupted 6-0 plain gut sutures.
- The lateral canthal tendon is repaired with a 4-0 Polyglactin suture placed in a loop fashion. The lateral canthal angle is reapproximated with a 6-0 plain gut suture; the remainder of the lateral canthotomy incision is closed with interrupted 6-0 plain gut sutures.

Immediate Postprocedure Care

Once the patient has been undraped and cleaned, a combination antibiotic/steroid ophthalmic ointment is applied to the eye and a monocular occlusive dressing is placed. The patient is taken to the postoperative recovery area and monitored before discharge. The authors prescribe a 7- to 10-day course of oral antibiotics. Over-the-counter analgesics (acetaminophen, nonsteroidal anti-inflammatory drugs) and oral narcotics typically offer good control of postoperative pain. Patients are scheduled for a postoperative visit the following day and given instructions to leave their dressing in place until this appointment.

Rehabilitation and Recovery

There is no specific rehabilitation required after this procedure. The authors recommend that patients resume light physical activity on the day following surgery. Heavy lifting (greater than 10 lbs) and strenuous activity should be avoided for 1 or 2 weeks. Patients should avoid activities with a risk of orbital trauma for at least 1 month.

Follow-up: Potential Complications and Their Management

A major goal of the 1-day postoperative appointment is to evaluate for the most serious and vision-threatening complication of any orbital surgery: a retrobulbar hemorrhage with optic nerve compression. Signs of this devastating condition include significant eye pain, proptosis, a "tense" orbit with increased resistance to retropulsion, decreased visual acuity, a relative afferent pupillary defect in the affected eye, and elevated intraocular pressure. Suspicion for this complication should prompt immediate intervention with lateral canthotomy and inferior cantholysis to decompress the orbit. Any delay in addressing this complication may result in permanent loss of vision. The authors have never encountered this rare complication after placement of an enophthalmic wedge implant and this is consistent with results in the literature.[25,26]

Other complications can be seen later in the postoperative period, most of which involve problems with the implant. Given the presence of a permanent foreign body in the orbit, there is always the possibility of developing an orbital infection. Mild infections may be treated initially with antibiotics. However, more severe infections, orbital abscess formation, or longstanding infections not resolving with antibiotics may

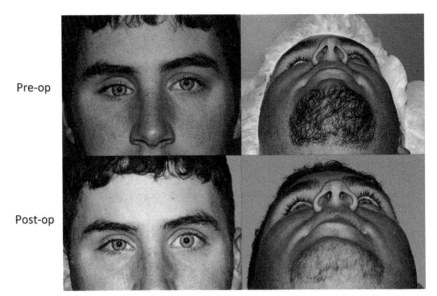

Fig. 5. Successful secondary repair of posttraumatic enophthalmos of the right eye using a high-density porous polyethylene enophthalmos wedge implant.

require surgical intervention with implant removal. Surgery is also indicated if an infection is associated with implant migration, exposure, or extrusion.

Furthermore, inappropriate implant positioning or sizing may result in extraocular muscle impingement, leading to diplopia or pain with eye movement. Management of this complication is surgical with orbital re-exploration and implant repositioning or exchange.

With the exception of retrobulbar hemorrhage, which requires immediate intervention, evaluation of these complications should include orbital imaging before deciding on the best approach to management.

Table 1
A brief literature review of high-density porous polyethylene wedge implants

Title	Pt Population	Pt #	Results
High-density porous polyethylene wedge implant in correction of enophthalmos and hypoglobus in seeing eyes[25]	Post-traumatic enophthalmos and hypoglobus	25	95.8% with improvement of enophthalmos 94.74% with improvement of hypoglobus No complications
Use of enophthalmic implants in the repair of orbital floor fractures[26]	Long-standing orbital floor fractures with enophthalmos, hypoglobus, and diplopia (3 of 4 patients) in primary position and downgaze	4	100% with resolution of enophthalmos and hypoglobus 100% with correction of diplopia in primary position with only mild residual diplopia in extreme upgaze No complications

Outcomes and Clinical Results in the Literature

Patients routinely do well after placement of an enophthalmic wedge implant with low rates of complications. The authors have had very good success with their patients with regard to secondary correction of enophthalmos (**Fig. 5**). In a review of 2 studies investigating the use of enophthalmic wedge implants as primary surgical treatment, greater than 95% of patients had successful correction of their facial asymmetry (**Table 1**).

SUMMARY

Enophthalmos is a frequent finding in the setting of facial trauma. When patients present with persistent clinically significant enophthalmos after primary repair of orbital fractures, an enophthalmic wedge implant is an effective surgical option if repair is deemed necessary.

REFERENCES

1. Bite U, Jackson IT, Forbes GS, et al. Orbital volume measurements in enophthalmos using three-dimensional CT imaging. Plast Reconstr Surg 1985;75:502–8.
2. Clauser L, Galiè M, Pagliaro F, et al. Posttraumatic enophthalmos: etiology, principles of reconstruction, and correction. J Craniofac Surg 2008;19:351–9.
3. Nolasco FP, Mathog RH. Medial orbital wall fractures: classification and clinical profile. Otolaryngol Head Neck Surg 1995;112:549–56.
4. Burm JS, Chung CH, Oh SJ. Pure orbital blowout fracture: new concepts and importance of medial orbital blowout fracture. Plast Reconstr Surg 1999;103: 1839–49.
5. Jank S, Schuchter B, Emshoff R, et al. Clinical signs of orbital wall fractures as a function of anatomic location. Oral Surg Oral Med Oral Pathol Oral Radiol Endod 2003;96:149–53.
6. He Y, Zhang Y, An J. Correlation of types of orbital fracture and occurrence of enophthalmos. J Craniofac Surg 2012;23:1050–3.
7. Koo L, Hatton MP, Rubin PA. When is enophthalmos "significant"? Ophthal Plast Reconstr Surg 2006;22:274–7.
8. Migliori ME, Gladstone GJ. Determination of the normal range of exophthalmometric values for black and white adults. Am J Ophthalmol 1984;98:438–42.
9. Manson PN, Clifford CM, Su CT, et al. Mechanisms of global support and posttraumatic enophthalmos: the anatomy of the ligament sling and its relation to intramuscular cone orbital fat. Plast Reconstr Surg 1986;77:193–202.
10. Kosaka M, Matsuzawa Y, Mori H, et al. Orbital wall reconstruction with bone grafts from the outer cortex of the mandible. J Craniomaxillofac Surg 2004;32:374–80.
11. Lee HH, Alcaraz N, Reino A, et al. Reconstruction of orbital floor fractures with maxillary bone. Arch Otolaryngol Head Neck Surg 1998;124:56–9.
12. Kontio RK, Laine P, Salo A, et al. Reconstruction of internal orbital wall fracture and iliac crest free bone graft: clinical, computed tomography, and magnetic resonance imaging follow-up study. Plast Reconstr Surg 2006;118:1365–74.
13. Cavusoglu T. Reconstruction of orbital floor fractures using autologous nasal septal bone graft. Ann Plast Surg 2010;64:41–6.
14. Cieslik T, Skowronek J, Cieslik M, et al. Bone graft application from anterior sinus maxillary wall in orbital floor reconstruction. J Craniofac Surg 2009;20:512–5.
15. Goiato MC, Demathe A, Suzuki T, et al. Management of orbital reconstruction. J Craniofac Surg 2010;21:1834–6.

16. Ng SG, Madill SA, Inkster CF, et al. Medpor porous polyethylene implants in orbital blowout fracture repair. Eye 2001;15:578–82.

17. Ozturk S, Sengezer M, Isik S, et al. Long-term outcomes of ultra-thin porous polyethylene implants used for reconstruction of orbital floor defects. J Craniofac Surg 2005;16:973–7.

18. Yilmaz M, Vayvada H, Aydin E, et al. Repair of fractures of the orbital floor with porous polyethylene implants. Br J Oral Maxillofac Surg 2007;45:640–4.

19. Jia-jie X, Li T, Xiao-lei J, et al. Porous polyethylene implants in orbital blow-out fractures and enophthalmos reconstruction. J Craniofac Surg 2009;20:918–20.

20. Garibaldi DC, Iliff NT, Grant MP, et al. Use of porous polyethylene with embedded titanium in orbital reconstruction: a review of 106 patients. Ophthal Plast Reconstr Surg 2007;23:439–44.

21. Gierloff M, Seeck GK, Springer I, et al. Orbital floor reconstruction with resorbable polydioxanone implants. J Craniofac Surg 2012;23:161–4.

22. Nam SB, Bae YC, Moon JS, et al. Analysis of the postoperative outcome in 405 cases of orbital fracture using 2 synthetic orbital implants. Ann Plast Surg 2006;56:263–7.

23. Imola MJ, Ducic Y, Adelson RT. The secondary correction of post-traumatic craniofacial deformities. Otolaryngol Head Neck Surg 2008;139:654–60.

24. Grus JS. Craniofacial osteotomies and rigid fixation in the correction of post-traumatic craniofacial deformities. Scand J Plast Reconstr Surg Hand Surg Suppl 1995;27:83–95.

25. Kashkouli MB, Pakdel F, Sasani F, et al. High-density porous polyethylene wedge implant in correction of enophthalmos and hypoglobus in seeing eyes. Orbit 2011;30:123–30.

26. Kempster R, Beigi B, Galloway GD. Use of enophthalmic implants in the repair of orbital floor fractures. Orbit 2005;24:219–25.

27. Mazzoli RA, Raymond WR, Ainbinder DJ, et al. Use of self-expanding, hydrophilic osmotic expanders (hydrogel) in the reconstruction of congenital clinical anophthalmos. Curr Opin Ophthalmol 2004;15:426–31.

28. Bacskulin A, Vogel M, Wiese KG, et al. New osmotically active hydrogel expander for enlargement of the contracted anophthalmic socket. Graefes Arch Clin Exp Ophthalmol 2000;238:24–7.

29. Schittkowski MP, Guthoff RF. Injectable self inflating hydrogel pellet expanders for the treatment of orbital volume deficiency in congenital microphthalmos: preliminary results with a new therapeutic approach. Br J Ophthalmol 2006;90:1173–7.

30. Vagefi MR, McMullan TF, Burroughs JR, et al. Injectable calcium hydroxylapatite for orbital volume augmentation. Arch Facial Plast Surg 2007;9:439–42.

31. Kotlus BS, Dryden RM. Correction of anophthalmic enophthamos with injectable calcium hydroxylapatite (Radiesse). Ophthal Plast Reconstr Surg 2007;23:313–4.

32. Vagefi MR, McMullan TF, Burroughs JR, et al. Orbital augmentation with injectable calcium hydroxylapatite for correction of postenucleation/evisceration socket syndrome. Ophthal Plast Reconstr Surg 2011;27:90–4.

Improving Posttraumatic Facial Scars

Farhad Ardeshirpour, MD*, David A. Shaye, MD,
Peter A. Hilger, MD

KEYWORDS

- Facial scars • Scar revision • Z-plasty • W-plasty • Geometric broken line closure
- Dermabrasion • Resurfacing • Camouflage

KEY POINTS

- Traumatic scars can aesthetically, functionally, and psychologically impair patients. Through comprehensive evaluation and thorough planning, patients should be counseled on realistic expectations.
- Fortunately, there are many surgical and nonsurgical techniques to greatly improve scars at several time points along the scarring process.
- Meticulous execution and postoperative care are necessary to achieve the best results.

INTRODUCTION

Posttraumatic facial scarring can be limiting from both physiologic and psychological standpoints. Some scars result in physical limitations to basic functions such as vision or eating. Others are simply an unpleasant reminder of a traumatic event of the past. Improving both function and aesthetics related to posttraumatic scarring are important goals in their treatment.

In the preoperative setting it is important to delineate the goals and expectations of scar revision. Patients often present with considerable misperceptions about what is feasible in scar revision. While decreasing the visibility of scarring is a reasonable objective, patients should be reminded that total elimination of a scar is not feasible. Moreover, recurrence of the same scarring pattern after repair can be an unfortunate possibility.

PREVENTION

The appropriate management of facial soft-tissue injuries begins in the acute setting. Foreign debris should be removed and wounds should be thoroughly irrigated to

Department of Otolaryngology, Head and Neck Surgery, University of Minnesota, 420 Delaware Street Southeast, Minneapolis, MN 55455, USA
* Corresponding author. Department of Otolaryngology, University of Minnesota, 420 Delaware Street Southeast, MMC 396, Minneapolis, MN 55455.
E-mail address: ardes003@umn.edu

Otolaryngol Clin N Am 46 (2013) 867–881
http://dx.doi.org/10.1016/j.otc.2013.06.006
0030-6665/13/$ – see front matter © 2013 Elsevier Inc. All rights reserved.

reduce bacterial counts. Conservative debridement can decrease the degree of persistent scarring and traumatic tattooing. The undermining of adjacent tissue may assist in the closure; however, elaborate flaps at the time of initial repair are usually inappropriate. Meticulous, tension-free closure in layers should be performed to minimize scar formation. Avoidance of infection through wound care and use of ointment or occlusive dressing optimizes healing. Posttraumatic infections are rare in the well-vascularized head and neck region. The literature shows that prophylactic antibiotics do not reduce infection rates but instead promote bacterial resistance. Prophylactic antibiotics have both increased cost and undesirable side effects (ie, diarrhea). Antibiotics should be reserved for patients with risk factors (ie, immunosuppression, diabetes), or wound risks (ie, animal bites, heavily contaminated wounds).[1] As in many surgical challenges, prevention is an important part of the overall treatment plan.

Wound Healing

The phases of wound healing must be considered to better understand the formation of facial scars. Would healing progresses through 3 phases: inflammatory, proliferative, and scar maturation/remodeling.[2] Youthful turgor can widen scars; the lack of facial rhytids also makes scars more apparent for a longer period. Conservative measures such as sun protection, intralesional steroid treatment for hypertrophic scars, and topical bleaching agents can all be essential parts of scar management. Discussing these issues with the patient at the initial consultation is an important part of the treatment plan.

Scar Physiology

Ideal scars are hidden, narrow, and flush with the adjacent skin. Prominent scars tend to have color mismatch, persistent erythema, and pigmentary irregularities (both hyperpigmentation and hypopigmentation). People with skin types higher on the Fitzpatrick Scale are more likely to have hyperpigmented scars. Those with lower Fitzpatrick skin types are more likely to experience persisting erythema and eventual hypopigmented scar. Contour irregularities can make scars more noticeable, particularly in direct overhead lighting. Textural abnormalities can also bring unwanted attention to a scar. Normal skin has a matte finish attributable to microsurface irregularities that scatter light. Scarring can lead to surface changes that alter these characteristics, resulting in a smooth surface and a shiny appearance.

The overall length of the scar is an important consideration. Scars up to 6 mm in length are often imperceptible, even if they do not follow the relaxed skin-tension lines. A long scar with a predictable direction is more noticeable, particularly those that do not follow the relaxed skin-tension lines. At a subconscious level, the eye is less drawn to scars that follow relaxed skin-tension lines. Facial motion increases the perceptibility of scars that run contrary to the relaxed skin-tension lines. Scars that lie along aesthetic subunit borders (ie, melolabial crease) or hide in natural shadows (ie, beneath the brow) are often less perceptible. By contrast, scars that are located over a prominence (ie, malar mound), particularly on a smooth, youthful face, are far more noticeable.

HYPERTROPHIC SCARS AND KELOIDS

Unlike light microscopy, scanning electron microscopy is able to show the difference between normal skin, hypertrophic scars, and keloids. Normal skin consists of distinct collagen bundles that run parallel to the epithelial surface. In comparison with normal skin, the collagen within hypertrophic scars are flat, wavy, less demarcated, and fragmented; however, collagen fibers of hypertrophic scars still run parallel to the surface.[3] The hypertrophic scar is confined within the borders of the wound, often occur in the early phases of injury, and may be erythematous, pruritic, and have telangiectasias. Hypertrophic scars are more likely to develop in areas of tension and are common with through-and-through injuries of the lip, particularly those that have some element of crush injury.

Keloids extend outside of wound borders and contain disorganized collagen fibers with random orientation to the surface. Keloids are more common in people with higher Fitzpatrick skin types and often occur in zones of increased tension, such as the clavicle, sternum, and upper back. Keloids in the face are a rare occurrence with the exception of the ear and neck.

Treatment of hypertrophic scars and keloids can include careful observation, camouflage, and revision surgery. For extensive facial scarring, custom-made pressure devices, as are often seen in burn units, may be considered. Laser technologies can also be used in the acute phases of scar hypertrophy to decrease vascularity and scar prominence. The most common and predictable treatment of scar hypertrophy is intralesional steroids. Dermal injections with triamcinolone acetonide (Kenalog; Bristol-Myers Squibb, New York, NY) at an initial concentration of 10 mg/mL can be used every 2 to 3 months as needed. Occasionally the concentration can be increased for recalcitrant lesions. Topical steroid application with flurandrenolide tape (Cordran Tape; Watson Pharmaceuticals, Corona, CA) or Silastic gel sheeting (Dow Corning Corp, Midland, MI) may also improve or prevent scars.[4] Aldara or 5% Imiquimod cream (3M Pharmaceuticals, St Paul, MN) is a topical immune-response modifier that stimulates an increase in collagen breakdown. The use of Imiquimod cream has prevented the recurrence of keloids after surgical excision in some studies, but further evaluation is needed.[5] Challenging scars are often treated with combination therapy, which can decrease the wound erythema and hypertrophy of dermal tissues.

Radiotherapy is typically reserved for scars that have failed other treatment modalities, but has been successful when combined with surgery. It has been postulated that radiotherapy limits collagen synthesis by altering fibroblast proliferation and inducing apoptosis. Many dosages and regimens have been described, but good results have been achieved with 15 to 20 Gy over 5 to 6 sessions in the acute postoperative period. Side effects include hyperpigmentation, erythema, and the rare but potential risk of radiation-induced malignancy.[5]

Physiologic Considerations

Structural distortion caused by a scar can alter physiology. For example, a scar that traverses the alar rim with subsequent scar contracture can result in nasal obstruction. Similarly, injuries near the eyelid or lip can cause retraction with ectropion formation or oral incompetence, respectively. Trauma to the scalp may cause telogen effluvium, and severe injuries may lead to permanent hair loss.

TREATMENT GOALS AND PLANNED OUTCOMES

For certain scars, medical and topical therapy alone does not achieve the desired result. When considering scar revisions, there are several patient characteristics that can influence treatment choices and timing:

- Age of the scar
- Age of the patient
- Skin pigmentation

- Multiple scars
- Patient education

Age of the Scar

The age of the scar is an important consideration. Surgical intervention in the inflammatory and proliferative phases may actually increase the total amount of scar-tissue formation. Thus, deferring surgery until scars have matured is often a prudent choice. In fact, scar maturation may significantly improve some of the previously discussed scar characteristics and obviate surgical treatment completely.

Age of the Patient

Patient age is also an important consideration. Tissue in younger patients is under greater tension, and relaxation of this tension is an important consideration before planning surgery. The age of the patient also influences the setting for revision. What can be a simple office procedure in an adult may necessitate general anesthesia in a child. Furthermore, functional loss has a significant influence on the timing of surgery. A scar contracture in the eyelid that creates an ectropion and corneal exposure mandates more urgent surgical intervention.

Skin Pigmentation

Skin pigmentation as represented by the Fitzpatrick Scale is also a consideration in treatment choice. Patients with Fitzpatrick skin scores greater than III are far more likely to develop postinflammatory hyperpigmentation following resurfacing technologies. Similarly, erythema that is slow to resolve is seen in lower Fitzpatrick skin types and may improve with the passage of time. If the patient or family has a history of scar hypertrophy or keloid formation, this should be discussed with the patient and family before surgical treatment.

Multiple Scars

Unfortunately, many traumatic incidents create facial lacerations with multiple independent or interconnecting scars. In these circumstances, the entire scar-maturation process is protracted and adjacent scars influence excisional treatment options. For example, if there are several nearly parallel scars with contour irregularities, scar excision and reapproximation may be an appropriate treatment option. However, it may be most appropriate to treat the scars sequentially rather than simultaneously, as the excisional treatment of both scars may result in excessive wound tension.

Patient Education

Finally, it is important to have clear communication with the patient about expectations for scar camouflage that is feasible and the duration and number of planned treatments. A patient with unrealistic expectations requires education on these issues before any scar-revision surgery is entertained. Patient education is greatly aided by reviewing photographs of other patients in one's practice and their outcome.

PREOPERATIVE PLANNING AND SURGICAL TECHNIQUES

Surgical intervention is often considered 6 to 12 months after the initial injury, before which concealment can be performed with the use of makeup and camouflaging.[6] In the interim, the wound can be improved with treatment options such as silicone sheeting, gel, or bleaching agents for areas of posttraumatic hyperpigmentation. Depressed areas or irregular surfaces may benefit from injections of biological fillers for temporary improvement. Ideally, definitive soft-tissue augmentation during surgery avoids the ongoing need for fillers.

A variety of surgical techniques is available to improve scars. The simplest option available for scars within relaxed skin-tension lines is excision and meticulous repair. This technique is best used for scars that are wide, have significant surface irregularities or traumatic tattooing, and follow the relaxed skin-retention lines. Scar tissue should be excised with undermining and mobilization of adjacent tissue. The incisions should be closed in layers, and the superficial layer should be meticulously repaired with fine, monofilament, permanent, or 6-0 fast-absorbing gut sutures. A thin layer of antibiotic ointment is applied, followed by the use of antitension tape for 1 week up to 3 months, depending on the surgeon's preference and the tension on the wound. Prolonged use of antitension tapes is often not feasible for patients after the first week.

Z-Plasty

A Z-plasty is a useful technique for scar lengthening and realignment. A Z-plasty is positioned such that the central limb lies over the contracted scar and the tangential limbs are positioned to rest as close as possible to the relaxed skin-tension lines. This technique is also useful for enlarging contracted orifices such as the mouth or nostril. Z-plasties are used to lengthen contracted tissues such as the eyelid with ectropion or lagophthalmos, or a cheek contraction that distorts the lips. A Z-plasty is also useful for making long, easily perceived scars less visible by establishing an irregular pattern that is more difficult for the eye to follow. The technique is also useful for reorienting scars that run perpendicular to the relaxed skin-tension lines (**Figs. 1** and **2**).

When performing the procedure, the scar and any deeper hypertrophic scar are first excised. The flaps are then incised and the perimeter of the defect undermined to allow for tissue redraping. The flaps are then transposed and repaired with buried, absorbable, subdermal sutures that eliminate any wound tension and create slight skin eversion. Dermal sutures placed a distance from the wound can help reduce tension. Superficial skin closure is performed with a monofilament permanent suture or 6-0 fast-absorbing gut suture. In some areas, the wound can be closed with subdermal or interdermal absorbable sutures and then topical tissue glue, which can reduce suture-track marks.

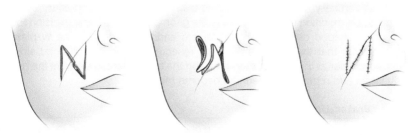

Fig. 1. Z-plasty technique used to reorient scar within the melolabial crease.

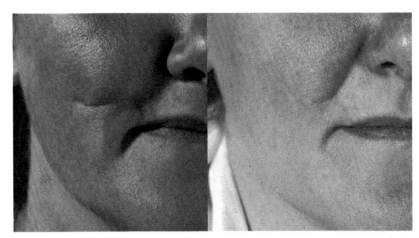

Fig. 2. A female patient who underwent Z-plasty to reorient her scar that was perpendicular to the melolabial crease. Reorientation along the facial subunits makes the scar less perceptible.

When designing a Z-plasty, first position the central limb of the Z over the axis to be lengthened which, in this discussion, is the central limb scar. The diagonal limbs lie relative to the relaxed skin-tension lines. The lengthening of scar increases with the measure of the angle between the central and diagonal limbs. Theoretically, a 30° angle results in a 25% lengthening of the scar; a 45° angle creates a 50% lengthening of the scar; and a 60° angle can generate a 75% increase in length (**Fig. 3**). The directional change of the central limb changes 90 degrees in a 60 degree z-plasty, 60 degrees in a 45 degree z-plasty, and 45 degrees in a 30 degree z-plasty. A Z-plasty of 60° causes excessive standing cutaneous cones. To optimally position the resultant scars along relaxed skin-tension lines it may be beneficial to design asymmetric angles along the Z-plasty. When possible, the Z-plasty should be designed so that the limbs are less than 1 cm in length. Larger scars are treated with multiple Z-plasties oriented along the length of the scar (**Fig. 4**). Although interesting from a mathematical perspective, compound Z-plasties have not been found to be clinically relevant.

W-Plasty

A W-plasty is another excisional treatment option that relies on breaking up a long, linear scar into multiple irregular segments. Limbs are kept under 6 mm to be less noticeable than those that are longer. The scar and underlying scar hypertrophy are resected, tissues undermined for at least 2 cm, and advanced into the area. This procedure permits the triangular tabs to interdigitate, thus breaking up the scar (**Fig. 5**). This technique is useful for scars that run perpendicular to the relaxed skin-tension line such as vertically up the forehead. It is also useful for an arced scar, for which the technique is modified to accommodate the geometry (**Fig. 6**). Scar excision results in a crescent-shaped defect with a longer arc and a shorter arc. The W-plasty is configured such that the triangles of tissue resected on the longer-arced side are considerably wider at their bases than those on the shorter-arced side. As the tissues are advanced and repaired, the lengths become more equal.

Geometric Broken-Line Closure

A geometric broken-line closure is a technique that was popularized by Dr Richard Webster in his practice in the 1960s and 1970s. This technique evolved from the

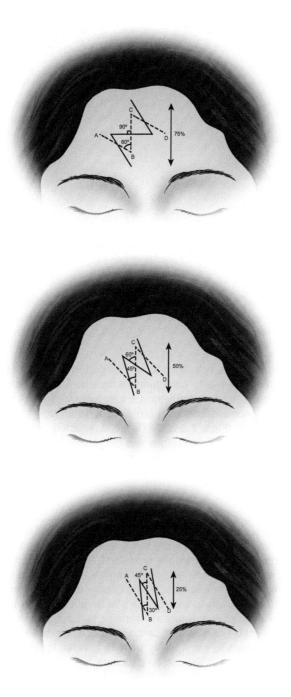

Fig. 3. In addition to reorienting scars, Z-plasties lengthen scars. The amount of lengthening correlates with the angle used to configure the Z-plasty. Larger angles between the central and peripheral limbs correspond with longer scars.

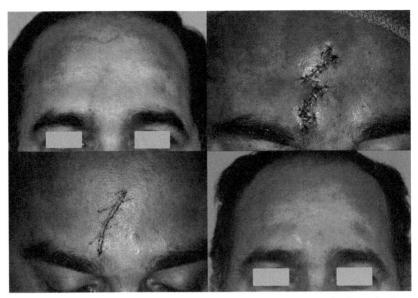

Fig. 4. A male patient with laceration to forehead who underwent multiple Z-plasties used to break up and reorient scar.

running W-plasty technique, but varied in that the pattern of excised tissue is irregular in nature. The running W-plasty configuration creates a predictable pattern that is more easily discerned. In the geometric broken-line closure, triangles, rectangles, and more complex geometric patterns are excised in mirror-imaged configurations on each side of the scar (**Figs. 7** and **8**). Tissue is resected, undermined, advanced, and repaired. Eversion of the skin edges and decreasing tension are important. The dermal layer can be closed with fine absorbable suture and skin repaired superficially with a running, locking, 6-0 fast-absorbing gut suture. Some surgeons also consider applying tissue glue to the surface.

Volume Issues

With all excisional techniques, soft-tissue volume alterations must be considered. Traumatic tissue loss or scar contraction may lead to depressions and other distortions that are more noticeable than the scar itself. These situations typically require consideration of volume replacement, which can be accomplished with several techniques. For example, when excising scar, the deeper dermal or fibrous elements can be retained and the surgically created flaps can be advanced over these tissues to enhance total volume. Liposculpture or transfer can accomplish the same result with meticulous injection of microfat parcels into deeper tissues. Biological fillers may also be considered to temporarily treat depressed or irregular areas. When volume excess occurs, the tissue can be debulked.[7]

RESURFACING

Resurfacing technologies can be used to camouflage minor contour irregularities. These irregularities can be the primary manifestation of the scar or persist after other excisional techniques. Resurfacing techniques include chemical peels, dermabrasion, and laser resurfacing. Chemical peels are most helpful on eyelid scars. Resurfacing

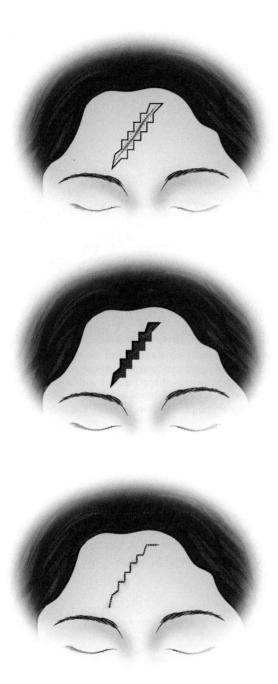

Fig. 5. Excision of scar using W-plasty technique, which makes the scar irregular and less noticeable. Some limbs of the W can be placed along the relaxed skin-tension lines. (*Data from* Westine JG, Lopez MA, Thomas JR. Scar revision. Facial Plast Surg Clin North Am 2005;13(2):328, vii.)

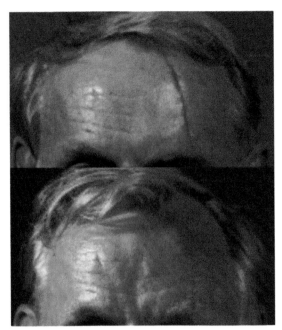

Fig. 6. A male patient with laceration to the forehead demonstrates how the W-plasty technique is useful for scars running perpendicular to the relaxed skin-tension lines of the forehead. Scar excision results in a crescent-shaped defect with a longer arc and a shorter arc. The W-plasty is configured such that the triangles of tissue resected on the longer-arced side are considerably wider at their bases than those on the shorter-arced side.

can be considered at any time from 6 weeks to 6 months after previous excisional techniques or after the initial injury itself (**Fig. 9**).[8]

Dermabrasion

Dermabrasion resurfacing is performed with an electric hand engine. Diamond fraise burrs of medium to coarse texture and a hand engine with both clockwise and counterclockwise rotation (speed of 35,000 rpm) are used. A local anesthetic is infiltrated and the surface is painted with gentian violet. Gentian violet is an effective antiseptic dye that flows into contour irregularities. The removal of the gentian violet can be a

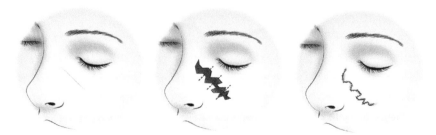

Fig. 7. Geometric broken-line closure technique excises the scar using different geometric designs, which irregularizes the scar. (*Data from* Westine JG, Lopez MA, Thomas JR. Scar revision. Facial Plast Surg Clin North Am 2005;13(2):328, vii.)

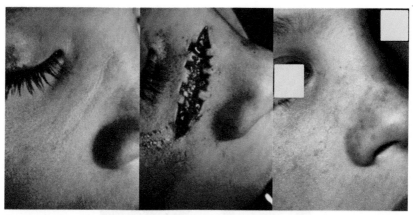

Fig. 8. A boy who underwent geometric broken-line closure of right nasojugal area, resulting in a more irregular and less noticeable scar.

guide to the depth of treatment (**Fig. 10**). Dermabrasion is performed until the papillary reticular dermal junction is visualized. More superficial resurfacing results in limited degrees of improvement. When performing dermabrasion, it is important that the surgeon and assistant wear appropriate protective garments.

Resurfacing is designed to lower the normal tissue to the level of the depressed scar. Raised hypertrophic scars or wide atrophic surface areas are unsuitable for resurfacing, because the skin appendages are necessary as an epithelial reservoir. Skin appendages are reduced in atrophic scars, and such resurfacing is avoided. Punctate bleeding indicates that the surgeon has reached the depth of the papillary dermis. When a fine, shredded appearance in the texture of the wound becomes

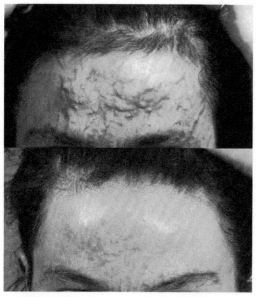

Fig. 9. (*Top*) A female patient who suffered from multiple forehead scars from lacerations 6 weeks previously. (*Bottom*) Results 3 weeks after dermabrasion.

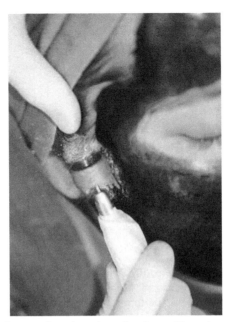

Fig. 10. A female patient undergoing dermabrasion with a drum-shaped fraise, which removes the gentian-violet dye painted on her face.

apparent, the superficial portion of the reticular dermis has been entered. Overly aggressive dermabrasion will remove tissue to a depth below the skin appendages, which results in increased scarring as the epithelium migrates from the periphery of the wound during healing.

Deeper penetration during skin resurfacing achieves effacement of contour irregularity. Conversely, this can increase the chance of pigmentary dyscrasias and reactive scar caused by dermal injury. Postinflammatory hyperpigmentation is a relatively common postoperative problem that is more evident in patients with a greater Fitzpatrick grade. Resurfacing of patients with a Fitzpatrick grade greater than III is generally avoided. Transient, postinflammatory hyperpigmentation often resolves with time and sun avoidance; however, the recovery period can be expedited by the use of bleaching agents. Hydroquinone and kojic acid are chemical agents that block the production of melanin, thereby decreasing postinflammatory hyperpigmentation. These agents do not remove the existing epithelial pigment but block the production of new pigment. Thus it takes 1 month to see the results of the bleaching agents because pigment migrates superficially as the epithelium is replaced from beneath. It is not uncommon to combine bleaching agents with topical corticosteroids to decrease the inflammation that provokes pigmentation. In addition, retinoids can be added to facilitate the removal of some of the epithelium and associated pigment, and increase the penetration of the other chemical agents. Sunscreens with a high sun protection factor and ultraviolet A/B coverage are an important adjunct to treatment, as postoperative sun exposure increases the likelihood of long-term pigmentary changes.

Postoperatively the wound is kept moist, as epithelial migration occurs more rapidly in a moist environment in comparison with wounds with crusts. The cleaning regimen includes regular cleansing of the wound with either half-strength peroxide or diluted vinegar solution (1 tablespoon of white vinegar and 8 ounces of water). These agents work well against skin pathogens. Topical antibiotic ointments are deferred, as there is a chance of provoking a contact sensitivity reaction, particularly with Bacitracin (Fougera & Co, Melville, NY).[9] To keep the wound moist a bland ointment such as Aquaphor (Beiersdorf Inc, Norwalk, CT) is used. Dressings are generally applied for the first 24 hours, then the wounds are left open and cleansed 4 to 6 times per day. It usually requires 7 to 14 days for the wounds to become reepithelialized, at which point camouflage makeup can be carefully applied. In the initial weeks after surgery the patient is instructed to use soapless cleansers, as the new skin is somewhat fragile.[10] Perioral resurfacing may activate latent herpes simplex eruptions, which may be prevented by prescribing suppressive antiviral therapy the day before surgery and continuing therapy until the wound epithelializes.

Laser

Carbon dioxide or Erbium laser resurfacing is another noninvasive option. More recently, the use of fractionated carbon dioxide lasers have produced excellent results. In a recent study by Jared Christophel and colleagues[11] fractionated laser resurfacing was compared with dermabrasion, and showed similar scar effacement. The fractionated carbon dioxide laser treatment is associated with decreased early postoperative erythema. For limited areas of superficial scarring over flatter, slightly convex surfaces, the use of dry-wall sandpaper has been shown to be effective.[12,13] The sandpaper can easily be cut into small segments and sterilized.

Areas of persistent erythema can be treated with a pulsed-dye laser, similar to that used in the treatment of congenital vascular anomalies. The treatments are spanned approximately 6 weeks apart. Acutely after treatment small ecchymotic lesions may appear, which are treated with conservative measures. There may be a small amount of epidermolysis, but this resolves well with conservative measures.

TISSUE EXPANDERS

When treating scars of moderate surface area, serial excision is a consideration. However, for larger areas tissue expansion is an excellent choice.[14] The forehead and scalp are excellent areas for use of tissue expansion. With expansion, the epidermis is expanded and thickened, with increased mitotic activity and decreased density of adnexal structures. The dermal thickness decreases during the expansion phase but returns to normal within 1 to 2 years. Placement of an expander adjacent to muscle results in decreased muscle thickness but without functional loss. Adipose cells decrease in number and subcutaneous thinning occurs. A capsule routinely forms around the expander, and angiogenesis increases flap viability. Bone remodeling can occur beneath the expander, but typically resolves over time. Certain anatomic areas are amenable to 2 expanders, which can decrease the overall treatment time.

Placement of the expanders is achieved by making incisions at the junction of the scar and normal tissue. A pocket is made in an avascular fascial plane, such as beneath the galea. The wound is closed in layers over the expander. Approximately 10% of the expander volume is added at the time of surgery to minimize the risk of hematoma formation around the expander. It is important to ensure that there are no wrinkles on the surface of the expander, which may cause pressure necrosis of the overlying soft tissues. Rectangular expanders with a base of approximately the same dimensions as the tissue to be replaced are selected. Expanders are inflated once or twice a week starting 2 weeks after placement. Patient discomfort or blanching over the surface of the expander is used as per treatment guidelines. It is important to overexpand the soft tissues, as there is some degree of contraction after removal. Any underlying bony contour changes are left untreated, as they resolve without any intervention. The capsule of the implant is left intact but is released along its margins. A 2-week hiatus is usually planned at the completion of expansion before the next stage of surgery, to allow the skin tension to decrease before flap creation. The character of the defect dictates flap design with the expanded skin. As mentioned earlier, 2 expanders are often used to decrease the length of expansion time. This approach also allows the design of complementary flaps for reconstruction (**Fig. 11**). The capsule of the flap is excised when a thin flap is desired. The flaps created have excellent viability as a result of the vascular changes that occur with expansion.

POTENTIAL COMPLICATIONS AND MANAGEMENT

Excision scar-revision techniques can result in flap compromise and loss of partial or full thickness. Aggressive resection can create undue tissue tension at the line of closure with the development of a wide atrophic scar or vascular compromise. Scar revision at the scalp can create transient or permanent alopecia. Contraction alopecia

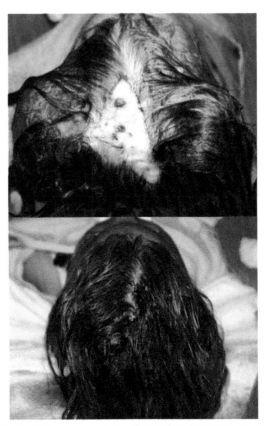

Fig. 11. (*Top*) A girl with 2 tissue expanders in her scalp adjacent to an area of congenital alopecia. (*Bottom*) Postoperative removal of tissue expanders and closure of elevated flaps.

is not uncommon, and resolves over a 3- to 4-month period. More extensive or permanent hair loss may necessitate tissue expansion or the use of hair transplantation. Caution must be used when working around hair follicles to avoid iatrogenic trauma with use of cautery or closure under high tension.

Hyperpigmentation can be treated with the use of bleaching agents as previously discussed for transient hyperpigmentation. More persistent pigmentation can be treated with laser technology, but again treatment of patients with a Fitzpatrick Scale greater than III can be challenging. Areas of tissue expansion or traction can develop telangiectasia, which if not resolving spontaneously can be treated with pulsed-dye laser therapy. Hypopigmentation can occur in areas of aggressive skin resurfacing or areas where there is excess wound tension, with widening of the scar and hypopigmented atrophic scar created. Hypopigmentation can be treated with either camouflage or reexcision, and advancement of healthier skin.

REFERENCES

1. Abubaker AO. Use of prophylactic antibiotics in preventing infection of traumatic injuries. Oral Maxillofac Surg Clin North Am 2009;21(2):259–64, vii.
2. Gosain A, DiPietro LA. Aging and wound healing. World J Surg 2004;28(3):321–6.
3. Atiyeh BS, Costagliola M, Hayek SN. Keloid or hypertrophic scar: the controversy: review of the literature. Ann Plast Surg 2005;54(6):676–80.
4. Kokoska MS, Thomas JR. Scar revision. In: Papel ID, editor. Facial plastic and reconstructive surgery. New York (NY): Thieme; 2009. p. 59–65.
5. Thomas J, Somenek M. Scar revision review. Arch Facial Plast Surg 2012;14(3): 162–74.
6. Sidle DM, Decker JR. Use of makeup, hairstyles, glasses, and prosthetics as adjuncts to scar camouflage. Facial Plast Surg Clin North Am 2011;19(3):481–9.
7. Shockley WW. Scar revision techniques. Operative Techniques in Otolaryngology-Head and Neck Surgery 2011;22(1):84–93.
8. Brenner MJ, Perro CA. Recontouring, resurfacing, and scar revision in skin cancer reconstruction. Facial Plast Surg Clin North Am 2009;17(3):469–487.e3.
9. Smack DP, Harrington AC, Dunn C, et al. Infection and allergy incidence in ambulatory surgery patients using white petrolatum vs bacitracin ointment. A randomized controlled trial. JAMA 1996;276(12):972–7.
10. Surowitz JB, Shockley WW. Enhancement of facial scars with dermabrasion. Facial Plast Surg Clin North Am 2011;19(3):517–25.
11. Jared Christophel J, Elm C, Endrizzi BT, et al. A randomized controlled trial of fractional laser therapy and dermabrasion for scar resurfacing. Dermatol Surg 2012;38(4):595–602.
12. Emsen IM. An update on sandpaper in dermabrasion with a different and extended patient series. Aesthetic Plast Surg 2008. [Epub ahead of print].
13. Poulos E, Taylor C, Solish N. Effectiveness of dermasanding (manual dermabrasion) on the appearance of surgical scars: a prospective, randomized, blinded study. J Am Acad Dermatol 2003;48(6):897–900.
14. Hoffmann JF. Tissue expansion in the head and neck. Facial Plast Surg Clin North Am 2005;13(2):315–24.

Facial Transplantation for Massive Traumatic Injuries

Daniel S. Alam, MD[a],*, John J. Chi, MD[b]

KEYWORDS

- Facial transplantation • Head and neck reconstruction • Microvascular surgery
- Neuromuscular reconstruction • Soft tissue reconstruction • Facial trauma

KEY POINTS

- The difficulty of facial reconstruction is in the complexity of the facial structures and functions.
- Conventional microsurgical reconstruction alone cannot effectively provide a neuromuscular reconstruction of significant facial defects, because there is currently no method to connect these reconstructions to the patient's motor cortex.
- Facial transplantation allows a composite transfer of skin, soft tissue, and bone that replaces the lost tissue with an exact anatomic and functional match.

INTRODUCTION

Facial reconstruction has made considerable progress over the last century. Injuries and defects that were once considered impossible to reconstruct have become amenable to modern techniques that are now considered standard of care. The evolution has seen an advance from the early developments of local soft tissue flaps and rigid fixation in reconstruction to the advent of microsurgical free tissue transfer. Complex three-dimensional facial defects can now be repaired using these free flaps. This development has allowed clinicians to not only coapt the residual tissue but also effectively replace significant amounts of tissue that is missing. From the early reports of free flaps in the 1980s to the complex reconstructions of the present day, flaps have undergone their own evolution. Time has made the extraordinary become ordinary. Flaps can be molded, prelaminated, and modified extensively to allow better reconstructions in this patient population. Despite all of these advances, there are certain defects and injuries that are encountered in clinical practice that still remain difficult challenges.

Financial Disclosures: None.
Conflict of Interest: None.
[a] Section of Facial Plastic & Reconstructive Surgery, Lerner School of Medicine, Head & Neck Institute, Cleveland Clinic Foundation, Case Western Reserve University, Desk A71, 9500 Euclid Avenue, Cleveland, OH 44195, USA; [b] Division of Facial Plastic & Reconstructive Surgery, Washington University School of Medicine, St. Louis, Missouri, USA
* Corresponding author.
E-mail address: alamd@ccf.org

Otolaryngol Clin N Am 46 (2013) 883–901
http://dx.doi.org/10.1016/j.otc.2013.06.001

LIMITATIONS OF CONVENTIONAL RECONSTRUCTION

The difficulty of facial reconstruction is in the intrinsic complexity of the face both in form and function. The face is composed of unique three-dimensional structures consisting of a wide variety of tissue types. The variation sometimes makes identification and transfer of appropriate donor tissue to this area challenging. The unique skin color, texture, and consistency of facial skin are often best reconstructed from adjacent areas within the face. Skin from distal extremities, although effectively transferred through microvascular techniques, is often not appropriately color matched to the face and becomes easily noticeable in the patient. The face also has unique structures that bear no similar homologues in other parts of the body, such as eyelashes and eyelids. The complex spatial relationships and varied tissue types of facial components, such as the nasal base to the upper lip and the junction of the red and white lip at the vermilion, create reconstructive challenges that are not easily overcome. Microvascular reconstruction of the face with the best outcomes is usually seen in cases of complex subcutaneous and bony reconstruction in which the skin and superficial musculoaponeurotic system envelope of the face is unaffected by the injury or surgical resection. When the neuromotor components of the face or facial skin are missing, the reconstruction of these areas becomes more difficult using conventional techniques, because harvest sites do not exist. Flap modification and revision can allow a progressive molding of the tissue to better approximate the desired end points, but there are limitations to this approach.

The difficulties in achieving the form of the face given its complexity, although daunting, are not the most significant limitation to conventional reconstruction. Repair of function is a bigger obstacle. Free flaps (with few exceptions) are static structural tissue transfers. Any motor function is caused by residual muscle function in the face. An example is a mandibular reconstruction with a fibula flap that relies on native function of the muscle of mastication to work. The face moves under complex discrete neuromuscular orders directing all of its activity: smiling, laughing, eating, speaking, and blinking. The ability to communicate emotions with the facial functions has no substitute. Any successful reconstruction of the face from a functional standpoint can not be limited to a replication of form but also needs to make this essential connection to the brain. It is this movement of the central face that is the critical component of all of its functional roles. Almost every facet of human communication and socialization relies on this. At a more esoteric level, but probably as important, the central face is the window to human emotion. People express anger, joy, grief, and love through the subtle and delicates movements of this part of the face. Injuries to this area not only affect the individual who experiences them but affects all of those around them. However, although surgeons have become adept at moving bone, skin, and soft tissue from one region of the body to another, they are still limited in their ability to establish a functional neuromuscular reconstruction. The only widely used clinical application of a neuromuscular flap in the face is the gracilis muscle for smile reconstruction. Although the results are excellent for this indication, the limitations of this procedure are obvious. The gracilis muscle is used primarily to reconstruct only the muscular component of the face and requires the remaining soft tissues and other structures to be intact and uninjured to achieve optimal results. The procedure is in principle solely the replacement of the critical zygomaticus major and minor complex. However, other significant reconstructive challenges remain. How do surgeons reconstruct facial defects when the other facial muscles (orbicularis oculi and oris) are missing? What are the options when facial skin and soft tissue are also missing?

These challenging questions arise when the face is injured by ballistic trauma. The restoration of bony landmarks and closure of soft tissue wounds is often not possible because of the loss of viable soft tissue and bone. In addition, the inherently poor vascularity of the severely traumatized tissues that remain and the associated evolving tissue necrosis and infection makes a challenging situation worse. Primary repair of the injured tissues is rarely feasible because adequate viable tissue is no longer present locally. The paradigm must shift from the classic conceptions of injury repair to rebuilding. Successful restoration of form and function can only be achieved by recruiting tissues to rebuild the deficient structures of the face.

The treatment approach for extensive traumatic head and neck injuries has shifted away from delayed repair to early repair with local tissue and free tissue transfer reconstructions. Staged early definitive reconstruction allows fewer surgeries and shorter hospitalizations. The initial repair may involve some elements of healing with secondary intention or primary closure but usually requires early recruitment of healthy tissue into the face via local tissue rearrangement, pedicled regional flap, or free tissue transfer (anterolateral thigh flap, osteocutaneous fibula flap). Local tissue advancement with a cervicofacial flap can be used to reduce the soft tissue deficit and provide skin coverage. Although this flap brings healthier adjacent tissue into the defect, it is a randomly based flap and susceptible to vascular compromise and distal flap necrosis. Pedicled regional flaps (paramedian forehead flap, deltopectoral flap, latissimus dorsi flap) are supplied by a vascular pedicle allowing greater tissue viability and versatility. The paramedian forehead flap can be used for nasal reconstruction. The deltopectoral flap and latissimus dorsi flap can be used to reconstruct large skin defects of the neck, lateral face, and scalp.

The evolving success and reliability of microvascular surgery has led to the early use of healthy vascularized free tissue transfer for trauma reconstruction. The advantages of recruiting nontraumatized naive tissue for the reconstruction include a more physiologic restoration of function and a reduction in scar contracture. Free tissue transfer also allows the reconstruction of varying tissue defects (mucosa, bone, skin, soft tissue) with comparable vascularized tissue. The anterolateral thigh flap can be used to reconstruct large skin and soft tissue defects. The osteocutaneous fibula flap can be used to reconstruct orbitomaxillary and mandibular defects. Many of these cases are discussed elsewhere in this issue.

Although the results are excellent, a few important points must be emphasized. All of the cases shown do not have significant neuromuscular losses of the central face. As discussed, conventional microsurgical reconstruction alone cannot effectively provide a neuromuscular reconstruction of significant facial defects. The face can be thought of as having 2 distinct physiologic regions. Most of the face and neck is composed of fasciocutaneous structures that are easily amenable to microsurgical and conventional reconstruction. However, the central face has significant neuromuscular functions and uniquely complex structures that are distinct. This relationship is shown in **Fig. 1**. Here the traditional techniques are grossly inadequate.

THE IMPORTANCE OF THE CENTRAL FACE

The consequences of the limitations in facial reconstruction of the central face are magnified by the importance this area has for quality of life. The functional significance of the area is obvious. Much of human communication depends on the function of the lips and mouth. Labial sounds such as B and P are common in almost all languages and they cannot be articulated without lip function. The function of the orbicularis oris is critical for eating and drinking. Nasal function and form are important to establish a safe and

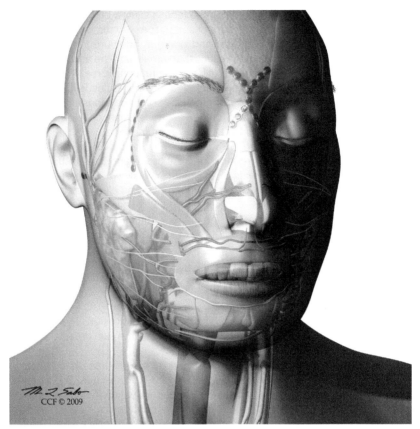

CCF © 2009

Fig. 1. The central neuromuscular face is shown in the colored segment. The static fasciocutaneous face is shown in black and white. (*Courtesy of* Cleveland Clinic Foundation, Cleveland, OH; with permission.)

appropriate airway. Eyelid function is critical for maintaining the ability to see. These functions represent just a few of the myriad vital functions that human faces play in daily life.

There are other reasons why midfacial injuries are so serious. The central face is also the key to people's physical identity. People are recognized more by the interplay of the structural relationship between the eyes, nose, and lips than any other part of the body. Within this small region, which is less than 5% of the body surface area, is the foundation of personal identity. This concept is illustrated in **Fig. 2**.

The high precision of human facial recognition is remarkable. Humans are able to distinguish more than 200,000 faces from each other. Within 50 hours of birth, newborn infants are able to recognize their own mothers from other individuals. The secondary consequences of this are profound. A mother shown images of her children activates rewards and socialization centers of the brain associated with feelings of positive emotions. These responses are unique and distinct from those seen when a mother is shown images of other children or strangers. The face offers the key to human connection. The bonds that are developed between friends and families are based on recognition of this critical region. There are data to suggest that the neurochemical relationships of human emotions are based initially on facial recognition and that this is the foundation for subsequent synaptic relationships to other centers of the brain.

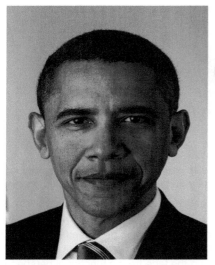 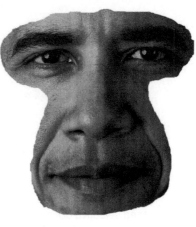

Fig. 2. (*Left*) The face. (*Right*) The central neuromuscular component that preserves the individual's identity.

Patients with significant midfacial injuries with severe disfigurement often claim that they think they are disconnected from society. The neurophysiologic data suggest that this is a problem that exists within the observer, not the injured patient. If someone does not have a face, it is almost impossible for observers to develop a normal human relationship with that person. Most patients who seek complex facial reconstruction with these types of injuries are not seeking a surgical procedure to return them to their preinjury state. They simply want to have the ability to return to human society.

THE RATIONALE FOR FACIAL TRANSPLANTATION

The complex movement of the midface and its critical importance to people's lives means that effective central facial reconstruction has to be a neuromuscular reconstruction. Simply replacing like tissue with like without reestablishing the connections to the brain results in a suboptimal masklike outcome. This result can be more disturbing than the defect itself. The movement of this area must be natural, with function that allows the patient to rejoin society. Because this cannot be recreated by borrowing tissue from another part of the patient's own body, the following question arises: what if surgeons were to use the same neuromuscular tissue complex from another individual?

The solution to this complex reconstructive challenge has been the use of allograft flaps. Facial transplantation has been used to reconstruct severe facial trauma injuries when massive loss of facial structures occurs. Although technically more challenging than the typical free tissue transfer and requiring lifelong immunosuppression for the recipient, face transplantation allows a composite transfer of varying skin, soft tissue, and bone that replaces the lost tissue with an exact anatomic and functional match.

Flaps have traditionally been viewed as the tissue that can be recruited within the angiosome of its pedicle vessel. To understand the rationale for facial transplantation, this concept needs to be extended to the idea of an angioneurosome. This concept is illustrated in **Fig. 3**. The design of the flap is based not only on the preservation of its blood supply but also on the concept of transferring a neuromuscular unit along with its muscular origin and insertion, including rigid facial structures and cutaneous ligaments. If this angioneurosome can be transferred in its entirety, it can be used

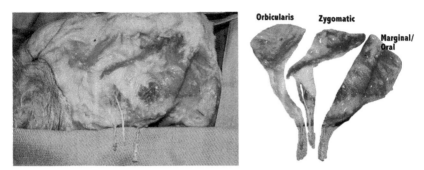

Fig. 3. The angioneurosome concept with the flap design based on preservation of vascular supply and transfer of a functional neuromuscular unit. (*Left*) The facial innervation. (*Right*) The individual functional regions.

to replace deficient tissue in a functional manner. Vascularization provides tissue viability, and then selective coaptation to the corresponding peripheral nerve restores movement and sensation. In doing so, clinicians have the option of not simply reconstructing a masklike facial form, but rebuilding the face from a functional perspective. For example, isolating each of the divisions of the facial nerve within an allograft specimen allows the surgeon to sequentially and segmentally rehabilitate the face.

MEDICAL RISKS

Facial transplantation procedures require a lifelong regimen of immunosuppression. This regimen can be associated with significant morbidity to the patient. A brief summary of the adverse effects and risks associated with this therapy is shown in **Fig. 4**. These risks must be weighed when considering the potential for this type of reconstruction.

Immunosuppression has been associated with an increased risk of cancer recurrences, as well as the development of new cancers. For this reason, a history of active cancer or a potential risk for recurrent tumor is an absolute contraindication at this time for allograft procedures, which are reserved within the context of experimental protocols at this juncture.

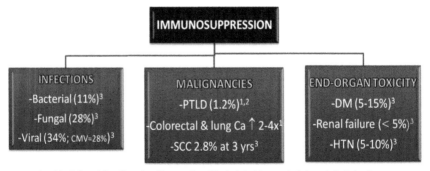

1. Morris P, et al. Face Transplantation: a review of the technical, immunological, psychological and clinical issues with recommendations for good practice. *Transplantation* 2007; 83: 109-128
2. Wiggins OP, et al. On the Ethics of Facial Transplantation Research. *The Am J of Bioethics* 2004; 4(3): 1-12
3. Vasilic D, et al. Risk Assessment of Immunosuppressive Therapy in Facial Transplantation. *PRS* 2007; 120: 657

Fig. 4. Adverse effects and risks associated with immunosuppression. *Abbreviations:* Ca, carcinoma; DM, diabetes mellitus; HTN, hypertension; PTLD, post transplant lymphoproliferative disorder; SCC, squamous cell carcinoma.

Rejection, both acute and chronic, is a serious potential complication of any transplant procedure and can result in organ loss. With the face, this potential sequela is magnified in significance. Appropriate salvage plans and backup protocols are essential steps in planning such a procedure. To date, there have been no faces lost because of rejection in compliant patients. However, acute rejection is a common phenomenon reported with multiple events in every case in the literature, but these episodes have been managed by short-term immunomodulation in all of the cases with relative ease.

ETHICAL CONSIDERATIONS

The medical risks associated with transplantation highlight one of the unique factors that must be considered in weighing the appropriateness of the procedure. At this time, face transplants remain experimental surgery and ethical considerations have been, and should remain, paramount in the development of any protocol for this surgery. A full discussion of the ethical implications of this procedure warrants its own article and is beyond the scope of this discussion. However, the general principles of autonomy, beneficence, and nonmalfeasance, which form the foundations of the ethics of medicine, should be considered in every case. The concept of potentially life-threatening complications for a reconstructive surgery is a reality with this procedure. The benefits must be enough to outweigh this risk. Therefore, the surgery should only be considered in individuals who have had a loss in their quality of life that warrants the acceptance of these risks. Proper evaluation of the capacity of the recipient to make this decision, their understanding of the risks and benefits, and their potential compliance with lifelong therapy is critical.

Beyond this difficult decision of risk/benefit there are other considerations unique to facial transplantation. The concept of identity is at the heart of this procedure. Do the recipients lose their identities? Do the donors transfer their identities? Or is it both? The preclinical data with cadaver work, as well as the clinical experience, have shown this to be less problematic than was initially predicted. Although full-face transplants share similarities to the donor, variations in skeletal structure and facial shape result in the recipient's transplanted face assuming a composite appearance that is neither donor nor recipient in origin.

The recipient's identification with and connection to the new face is a transformation in itself. However, this has not been a difficult adjustment for patients to make. In their own words, they have lost their old faces and now are so disfigured that they feel inhuman. The goal in these patients is not to restore their preinjury faces, but merely to have faces that allow them to return to human socialization. In many respects, this represents a paradigm shift for the reconstructive surgeon whose holy grail has always been the restoration of the preinjury state. Facial transplantation is not restoration, it is replacement.

SURGICAL INDICATIONS FOR FACIAL TRANSPLANTATION

Facial transplantation should be reserved for individuals with significant midfacial neuromuscular injuries. Complete absence or loss of the function of the orbicularis oris muscle along with a concurrent complete nasal defect is probably the minimal indication for considering allograft-based reconstructions. Defects can extend beyond these limits to include eyelids and the full face, but the minimum deficit requiring allograft approaches is the central neuromuscular segment of the midface. The inclusion criteria at present include ballistic and physical trauma (ie, burns) exclusively. The potential risk of the loss of cancer surveillance under immunosuppression precludes postsurgical ablation of malignancy as a potential indication.

ALLOGRAFT DESIGN AND CLASSIFICATION SCHEME

Numerous allograft procurement protocols have been described in the literature. At this early stage of the procedure, most allografts have been tailored to the defects of the individual patients. At the time of writing of this article, only 25 facial transplantation procedures have been performed worldwide. Despite the variability in the cases, some common themes are present across all of the procedures. The facial artery alone provides the arterial inflow in most (18 of 25) cases, and in a few cases the external carotid artery has been used. Angiographic studies, as well as clinical experience, have shown that the facial artery is sufficient to supply a full-face transplant including the maxilla. Although primarily supplied by palatine vessels from the internal maxillary system, the palate can easily be perfused via oral mucosal vascular networks from the facial artery. The venous outflow has traditionally been based on the common facial veins, as well as the external jugular venous system. Some surgeons have chosen to use the internal jugular vein, but the common facial vein is adequate for the venous drainage of the inferior facial structures. The cross circulation in the face is so well established that vascular reconstitution of one side of the face alone allows perfusion of both sides across the midline.

The depth of the allograft harvest must be below the plane of the facial musculature and the facial nerve. In order to achieve a neuromuscular reconstruction, the facial nerve must be carefully dissected and preserved. Individual facial nerve branches are isolated and a sequential and segmental series of neurorrhaphies is performed.

A simplistic way to understand the various facial procurement protocols is to consider them as a combination of traditional surgical approaches. For example, the combination of a bicoronal flap, a Le Fort 3 level osteotomy, and bilateral superficial parotidectomy plan elevation is a full-face procurement. The bicoronal flap, which is a component of all facial procurement protocols, and the other surgical approaches used preserve allograft vascularity and nerve function. Using a combination of surgical approaches a blueprint for the allograft procurement appropriate for the patient's facial defects can be created. The procurement procedures are not novel surgical techniques, but merely a new perspective on the use of accepted surgical approaches.

CLINICAL EXPERIENCE

At this early point in the history of facial transplantation, the worldwide clinical experience is too limited to have any significant data to support its long-term efficacy. The largest reported clinical series remains only 3 patients. Thus, the reports remain an exercise in proof of concept and anecdotal experience. My personal involvement in facial transplantation has involved 2 cases. I was the primary surgeon for the first case in the United States (case #4 worldwide), involving a patient with a shotgun injury to the midface. I was also a part of the surgical team for a second patient who had injury from an animal attack resulting in a total facial avulsion and who underwent a full-face transplant (case #21 worldwide). The evolution of this surgical procedure during the time between these two cases shows the rapidly advancing nature of this field.

Case 1

Indication
At the time of her facial transplantation, this patient was a 46-year-old woman who had undergone 23 prior reconstructive procedures, including 4 failed free flaps performed by an outside group of surgeons. Her preoperative clinical presentation is shown in **Fig. 5**. She continued to have significant disfigurement and functional limitation after

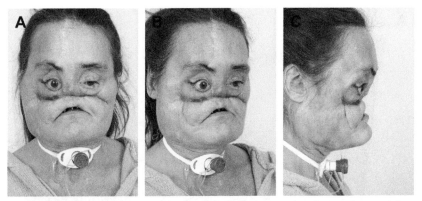

Fig. 5. (A–C) Preoperative clinical presentation of the first US facial transplant recipient.

these procedures and therefore was seen for evaluation by the multidisciplinary Cleveland Clinic Face Transplant Team (established in 2004 following institutional review board approval).

The midface of this patient was functionally absent or surgically altered. The extent of the defect included the absence of any nasal or septal structure. This defect had been previously managed by soft tissue coverage using a paramedian forehead flap. There was also an absence of maxilla, zygomatic arches, and inferior orbital rims. In addition, scar contracture in the midface and the prior flap coverage eliminated a nasal passageway, rendering the patient anosmic and an obligate mouth breather. The absence of any mimetic musculature in the midface left her with a functional bilateral facial paralysis and significant oral incompetence. The tissues in this region were residual components of her prior reconstructions and were nonfunctional. Another consequence of her extensive prior surgeries was scarring and fibrosis in the soft tissue of the neck and the resultant depletion of suitable recipient vessels.

Anatomic design and flap procurement

Based on the specific anatomic requirements of this patient, the technical design of the donor flap was undertaken once the exhaustive pretransplant work-up was finalized. This pretransplant assessment included evaluations from the departments of transplant surgery, transplant psychiatry, and bioethics. The complex nature of the patient's skeletal loss presented the unique challenge of incorporating vascularized maxilla into the transplanted face. The design of the donor facial soft tissue and skin envelope incorporated the cheek subunit, the nose, and the upper lip. The flap was planned as a full-thickness flap including the buccal mucosa of the midface. In the lower third of the face, where the patient had existing viable tissue, the allograft flap was procured in the subplatysmal plane with incorporation of both the parotid and portions of the submandibular glands for safe preservation of the neurovascular pedicles. This design intentionally incorporated redundant glandular tissue, which will need to be removed in a planned revision procedure in the future. The donor's hypoglossal nerves were also included as a motor nerve graft to bridge the gap between the recipient's midface division branch of the facial nerve and the donor facial nerve trunk created by the redundant parotid gland tissue. Because the inflow axons are only midface in origin, this neurorrhaphy reduces potential synkinesis and inappropriate facial movement. The transplant allograft is shown in **Fig. 6**. The surgical steps are outlined in **Fig. 7**.

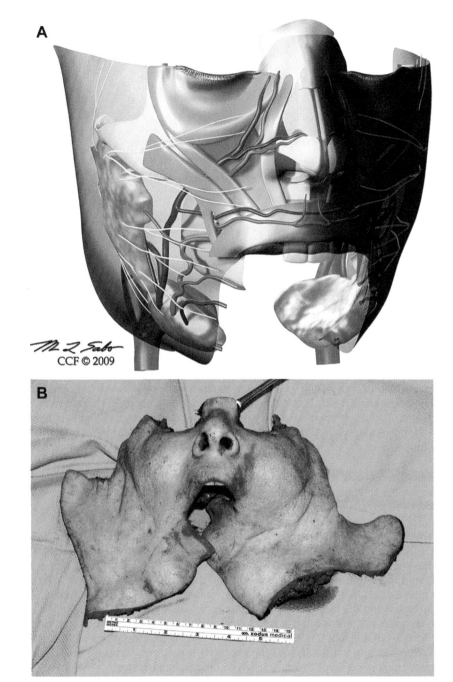

Fig. 6. The facial transplant allograft (*A*) Schematic. (*B*) The specimen. ([*A*] *Courtesy of* Cleveland Clinic Foundation, Cleveland, OH; with permission.)

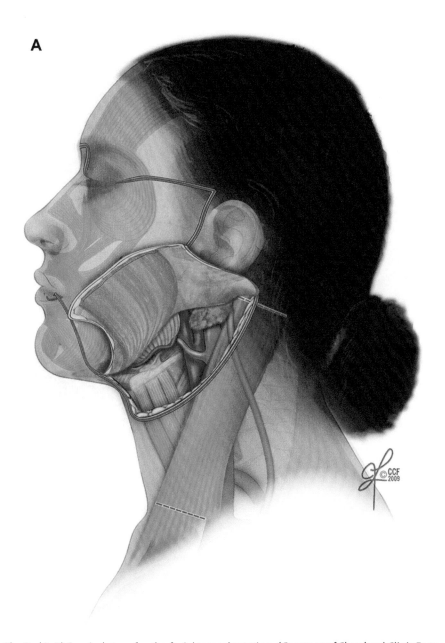

Fig. 7. (*A–D*) Surgical steps for the facial transplantation. (*Courtesy of* Cleveland Clinic Foundation, Cleveland, OH; with permission.)

B

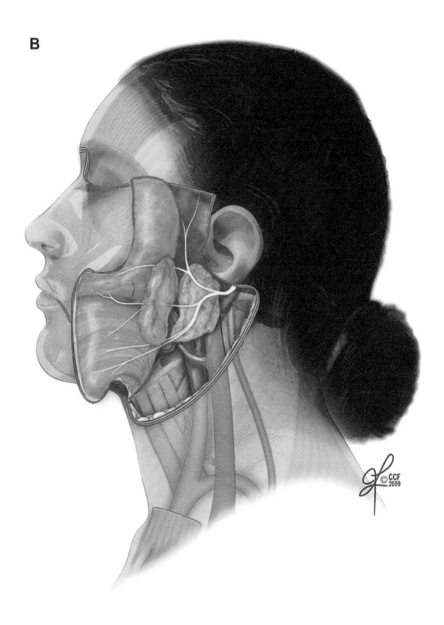

Fig. 7. *(continued)*

C

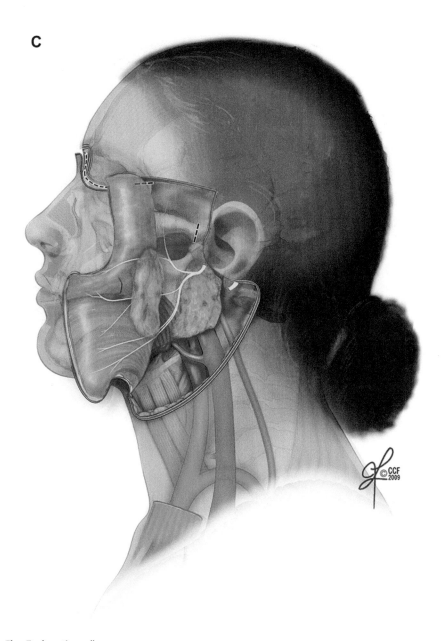

Fig. 7. *(continued)*

D

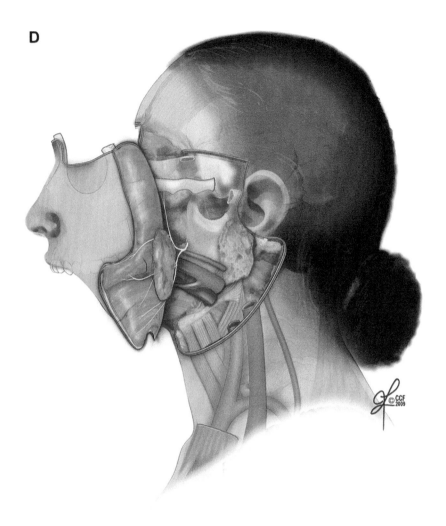

Fig. 7. *(continued)*

Outcomes

Late postoperative outcomes are shown in **Fig. 8**. At the time of the writing of this article, it is 4 years since the surgery. The incorporation of the allograft has been complete with no graft loss. She has recovered facial nerve function and facial sensation. She has had restoration of all of her midfacial functions that were lost following her injury, including smiling and laughing. The aesthetic outcomes are limited by her pre-existing eyelid trauma, which has not been addressed by the transplant, as well as the outcomes of the transplant itself. She has redundant parotid tissue that needs to be removed and her facial nerve has been asymmetric with greater functional recovery on her left side. Despite these limitations, she is able to integrate herself into social environments almost seamlessly.

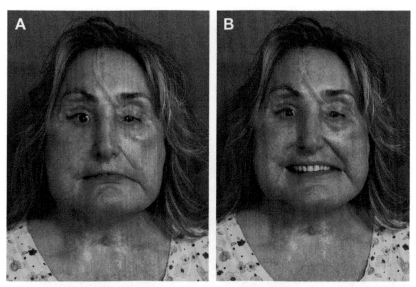

Fig. 8. Late postoperative outcomes (~4 years after facial transplantation), showing recovery of the facial nerve and midfacial function. *A* shows the Patient in repose and *B* shows the Patient smiling.

Case 2

Indication

At the time of her facial transplant, the patient was a 56-year-old woman who had been attacked by a chimpanzee, resulting in a near-total facial avulsion. She was initially managed with debridement and wound care to stabilize her infected wounds. At initial presentation, she was in a medically induced coma from which she was unarousable. She awoke approximately 1 month following her injury and regained normal cognitive function. She subsequently underwent interval recon-struction with local advancement flaps, an anterolateral thigh free flap, and rib carti-lage graft to temporize her condition. Her initial presentation and repair is shown in **Fig. 9**.

Anatomic design and flap procurement

The extent of injury in this case required a full facial transplant. Although the prior procedure was planned with the approach of defining a unique and novel surgical approach to the defect, the design of this transplant was based on traditional surgi-cal approaches. The design of this flap is shown in **Fig. 10**. The allograft is a com-posite of a bicoronal flap, bilateral parotid dissections, Le Fort 3 level osteotomies, and oral mucosal release. The neck plane is in the standard subplatysmal plane with dissection of the facial arterial and venous vascular system. The superficial pa-rotid glands are removed in this case, eliminating the need for revision parotid surgery.

With full facial transfer, isolation of individual facial nerve branches is a critical step. Neural coaptation was performed at distal locations to prevent synkinesis and to improve selective motor function. Patients with injury to the facial nerve proximal to the pes anserinus are poor candidates for full facial transplantations for this reason.

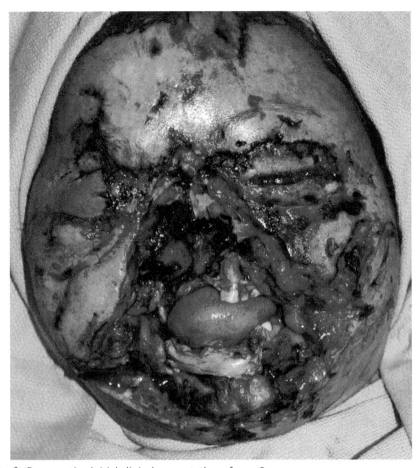

Fig. 9. Preoperative initial clinical presentation of case 2.

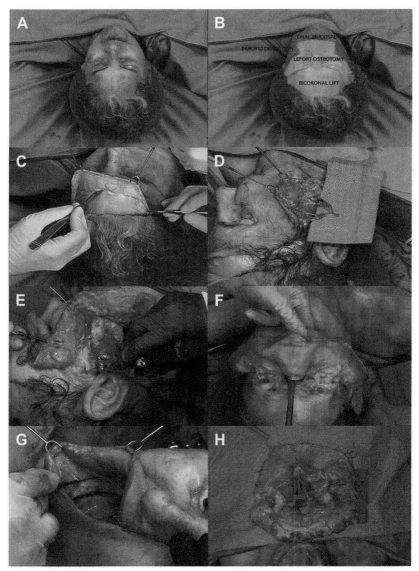

Fig. 10. (*A–H*) Full-face procurement: bicoronal flap, a Le Fort 3 level osteotomy, and bilateral superficial parotidectomy plane elevation.

Outcomes

The immediate postoperative outcome of this patient is shown in **Fig. 11**. She is now almost 2 years after transplantation, with full graft take and functional recovery. She has restoration of functional facial movement bilaterally, although her facial nerve function remains slightly paretic. She has been able to return to society, in spite of her blindness and loss of hands that remain significant residual disabilities.

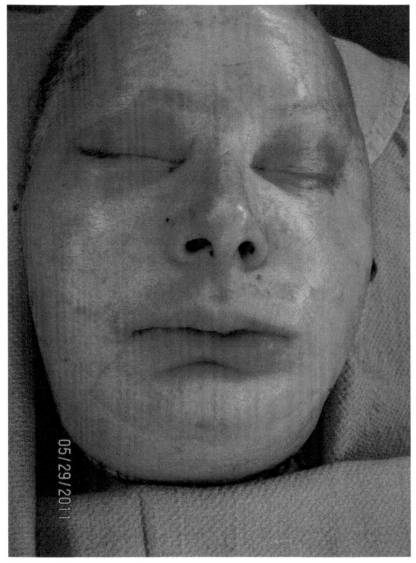

Fig. 11. Immediate postoperative outcome.

SUMMARY

Despite the early stage of facial transplantation, optimism for its role in facial reconstruction remains high. This optimism is the consequence of both the successful early outcomes and the complex nature of the problem that the surgery addresses. There is currently no way to repair complex neuromuscular injuries of the face. Although free flaps have offered an effective tool to transfer tissue, surgeons remain unable to functionally connect the transferred tissues to the brain to create a functional reconstruction. The gracilis free flap reconstruction begins to address this issue but it is a limited indication for a single function. In massive injuries, there are still no satisfactory options. It is in this futility that the strongest arguments in favor of facial transplantation can be made.

Over the first 25 cases, the technique has improved and this trend should continue as more cases are performed and long-term follow-up of early cases becomes possible. The success of this operation remains an unanswered question at this stage, but the early outlook remains promising.

SUGGESTED READINGS

Alam D, Papay F, Djohan R. Technical and anatomical aspects of the world's first near total face and maxilla transplant. Arch Facial Plast Surg 2009;11(6):369–77.

Alexander AJ, Alam DS, Gullane PJ. Arguing the ethics of facial transplantation. Arch Facial Plast Surg 2010;12(1):60–3.

Devauchelle B, Badet L, Lengele B, et al. First human face allograft: early report. Lancet 2006;368:203–9.

Dubernard JM, Lengele B, Morelon E, et al. Outcomes 18 months after the first human partial facial transplantation. N Engl J Med 2007;357:2451–60.

Guo S, Han Y, Zhang X, et al. Human facial allotransplantation: a 2-year follow-up study. Lancet 2008;372:631–8.

Lantieri L, Meningaud JP, Grimbert P, et al. Repair of the lower and middle parts of the face by composite tissue allotransplantation in a patient with massive plexiform neurofibroma: a 1-year follow-up study. Lancet 2008;372:639–45.

Lantieri L, Hivelin M, Audard V, et al. Feasibility, reproducibility, risks and benefits of face transplantation: a prospective study of outcomes. Am J Transplant 2011;11: 367–78.

Meningaud JP, Paraskevas A, Ingallina F, et al. Face transplant graft procurement: a preclinical and clinical study. Plast Reconstr Surg 2008;122:1383–9.

Pomahac B, Lengele B, Ridgway EB, et al. Vascular considerations in composite midfacial allotransplantation. Plast Reconstr Surg 2010;125:517–22.

Pomahac B, Pribaz J, Eriksson E, et al. Restoration of facial form and function after severe disfigurement from burn injury by a composite facial allograft. Am J Transplant 2011;11:386–93.

Siemionow M, Papay F, Alam D. Near total human face transplantation for a severely disfigured patient in the USA. Lancet 2009;374(9685):203–9.

Soni CV, Barker JH, Pushpakumar SB, et al. Psychosocial considerations in facial transplantation. Burns 2010;36:959–64.

Massive Traumatic Composite Tissue Loss

Application of Autologous Free Tissue Transfer in the Management of Massive Traumatic Tissue Loss

Michael A. Fritz, MD*, Timothy M. Haffey, MD

KEYWORDS

- Massive facial trauma • Free tissue transfer • Posttraumatic tissue loss
- Gunshot wounds • Microvascular reconstruction

KEY POINTS

- Free tissue transfer is a critical tool in the management of facial injuries with large composite losses and has led to substantial improvements in reconstructive outcomes.
- A management philosophy that follows a staged approach to accomplish structural replacement first followed by functional restoration and finally by aesthetic form serves as a valuable guide in surgical planning.

INTRODUCTION

Before the advent of free tissue transfer, management of extensive traumatic facial injuries was limited to locoregional techniques and secondary intention healing, often leading to significant tissue contracture and structural loss. As a result, severe functional and aesthetic deficits paralleled the overall degree of tissue loss. As surgeons' ability to reliably replace soft tissue and bone deficits with imported vascularized tissue has improved, the potential for favorable outcomes has increased exponentially. That being said, restoration of satisfactory form and function after massive facial trauma with significant tissue loss remains one of the most daunting challenges encountered by reconstructive surgeons.

In contrast to typical ablative facial defects due to tumor resection, there are particular issues in traumatic wounds that impart a greater degree of difficulty for the reconstructive surgeon. First, the initial traumatic defect is essentially tissue loss in evolution; as exposed, marginally vascularized, damaged, and contaminated tissue continues to die off for a period of time—this phenomenon is particularly relevant in

Department of Otolaryngology—Head and Neck Surgery, Head and Neck Institute, Cleveland Clinic Foundation, A71, 9500 Euclid Avenue, Cleveland, OH 44195, USA
* Corresponding author.
E-mail address: fritzm1@ccf.org

Otolaryngol Clin N Am 46 (2013) 903–913
http://dx.doi.org/10.1016/j.otc.2013.06.004
oto.theclinics.com

blast injuries (eg, close range gunshot wounds), which comprise a large number of these defects. Second, and nearly simultaneous with tissue loss, forces of healing contracture are often unopposed due to loss of underlying bone structure and opposing muscular function. This process creates wound distortion, pulling free soft tissue and bone into distorted, nonanatomic planes. Although continued contracture results in a smaller wound and apparently less future reconstructive need (rationale for allowing early secondary healing in the past[1,2]), this apparent benefit is deceptive, as it is gained at the expense of final functional and aesthetic outcomes. For these reasons reconstructive paradigms have evolved over time, and many authors argue for immediate definitive reconstruction after careful debridement.[3–5]

Evolving tissue loss, contracture, and granulation tissue result in a wound that is starkly different in appearance and behavior than the typical ablative defect encountered by reconstructive surgeons. The wound is distorted and typical landmarks (eg, contiguous mandibular structure) are absent to guide bone reconstruction. Nerves and vascular structures are obscured by traumatized tissue and scar and are often displaced from anatomic locations because of adjacent volume loss and contracture. Furthermore, elevation of fragile watershed tissue to achieve exposure for reconstruction often results in further loss of native tissue postoperatively.

TREATMENT GOALS AND PLANNING

The eventual goal of the reconstructive surgeon, as it always should be, is to restore function and form to the point of wound imperceptibility; however, particularly in this setting, it is often impossible to replace dynamic muscle, normal bone, soft tissue form, and color-matched skin. In contrast to smaller and more controlled reconstructions, it is exceedingly rare to achieve an optimal result in a single-stage operation. Therefore, a calculated, staged approach is required, analogous to large-scale reconstruction of cutaneous defects encountered after removal of large cutaneous malignancies (ie, "Mohs reconstructive mindset").

Three major goals in specific order provide a guide for reconstruction; these are

1. Replacement of structure
2. Restoration of function
3. Reestablishment of aesthetic form

Often, inroads toward these goals are made simultaneously, but attempts at the latter goals without fulfillment of the former will often undermine the final outcome.

Replacement of bone and soft tissue structure serves several roles, which optimizes final outcomes. Restoration of bone structure (eg, mandible, midface, orbit) allows for support and functional preservation of critical structures, such as the eye, lip, palate, and anterior tongue/airway. In the case of massive traumatic loss, free tissue transfer allows for replacement of like tissue in an unrestricted and untethered orientation, eventually allowing preserved muscle to function unopposed, providing the best opportunity for the patient to achieve a functional outcome, such as eye protection or oral competence (**Fig. 1**A–G).

Given the ample bone stock tolerant to structural modification and large soft tissue and skin components, fibula free tissue transfer is the most common and valuable technique in restoration of large composite losses.[6] Furthermore, fibula bone provides acceptable foundation for osseointegrated implants,[7,8] which are of paramount importance to achieve full rehabilitation in this typically younger and more active patient population. This full rehabilitation can be achieved during the primary[9] surgery, or as a secondary surgery. Scapular/parascapular flaps also carry advantages of composite tissue transfer with even more malleable cutaneous paddle orientations; however, this comes at the expense of bone stock and pedicle length. Additional commonly used techniques for soft tissue and cutaneous replacement include radial forearm and anterolateral thigh flaps; the latter is used preferentially given more abundant and malleable tissue, with less harvest site morbidity.

Before proceeding toward the first goal of structural replacement and obviously following initial patient stabilization (ie, bleeding and airway control), a period of observation/debridement is required to allow wounds to become quiescent and defined. In the case of close range blast injuries, serial trips to the operating room with wound cleaning and debridement are performed for approximately 3 weeks before definitive management, allowing for calculated surgical planning and minimizing die off of watershed tissues due to both clear tissue demarcation and revascularization of marginal regions.

In the first stage of structural replacement, the wound is fully defined and the remaining functional tissues (eg, lip elements) are released to preinjury anatomic positions. Critical bone and soft tissue are replaced to support functional tissue and provide a foundation for normal facial form and sufficient cutaneous coverage to prevent further contraction. In contrast to typical facial reconstructions, tissue color and volume mismatch are not relevant at this initial stage. These regions will be addressed as tissue is "sculpted" after it heals and softens.

Additional stages of reconstruction are performed after an interval period of wound healing and stabilization (see **Fig. 1**D–G). Typically 6- to 12-week intervals are required to achieve this goal, but examination and wound palpation are the most important factors influencing timing. In these stages, more traditional locoregional techniques (eg, circumoral myocutaneous flaps, myocutaneous eyelid transpositions) are combined with aggressive tissue undermining, flap transposition, and advancement to lengthen lip and eyelid height, remove color-mismatched skin, and create more appropriate contour (see **Fig. 1**; **Fig. 2**; see **Fig. 7**). Typically, retention of tissue bulk from free flaps is critical in regions of massive loss and only superficial elements are removed as advanced color-matched skin provides coverage. Serial surgeries of this nature with interval periods of tissue relaxation create a process analogous to slow tissue expansion and often allow for complete removal of initial color mismatched regions. These additional stages require cautious preservation of dermal/subdermal plexus connections to avoid compromise of blood supply. Both careful preoperative planning and a flexible intraoperative approach are key in obtaining success at this stage. Often, the surgical and technical challenge of modification of native and transferred tissues rivals initial structural replacement.

PATIENT EDUCATION AND MANAGING EXPECTATIONS

Detailed preoperative discussions with both patients and families are critical to provide a foundation of trust and to clarify expectations. It is important to review the series of goals (ie, structure, function, and form) specifically as well as the timing of additional revisions. Depending on injury sites and degree of tissue loss, functional and aesthetic compromise may be inevitable. Frank discussions in this regard are important but can be counterbalanced by emphasis on the reconstructive surgeon's long-term commitment to optimizing outcomes to buoy patient and family morale. In addition, given the frequency of native tissue loss at wound margins following initial structural replacement with free tissue transfer, it is wise to expect and predict this phenomenon in preoperative discussions. By having this discussion, evolving wounds are viewed as expected outcomes rather than complications. If patients and families understand

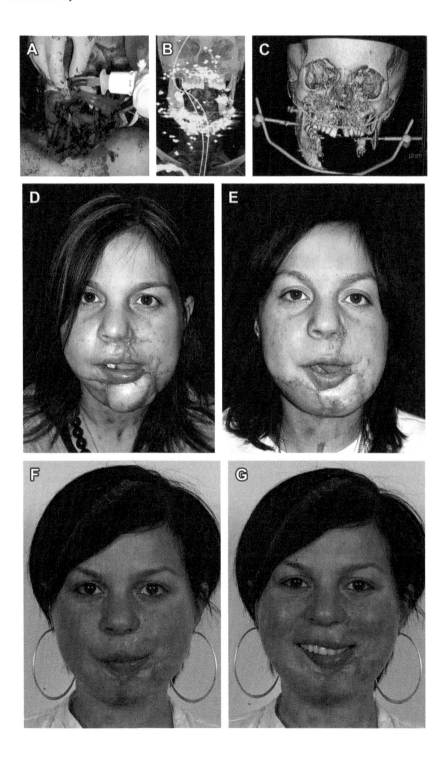

that their rehabilitation is a "marathon" with expected ups and downs, their tolerance of this difficult course is improved.

SITE-SPECIFIC APPROACHES AND CASE EXAMPLES

Concise discussion of massive traumatic tissue loss is difficult in that management essentially encompasses all aspects of major facial reconstruction depending on the subsites affected. After considering and adapting to the previously described differences in wound behavior and reconstructive philosophy, general reconstructive techniques with free tissue transfer are broadly applicable. Approaches to lower and mid facial reconstruction will be emphasized over cranial and skull base reconstruction as complexities of the latter are typically limited and vary little from general skull base reconstructive techniques (ie, free vascularized tissue to protect cranial structures and control cerebral spinal fluid leaks). In addition, many patients with major traumatic injuries involving the skull base and cranial structures do not survive initial injuries.

LOWER FACIAL LOSS

Lower facial loss is commonly encountered in blast injuries and self-inflicted gunshot wounds, due to both the position and the prominence of the mandible. The major goals of lower facial reconstruction are to restore mandibular continuity to achieve structural form, airway protection, and oromotor function and to establish a platform for dental rehabilitation. As previously outlined, this is most commonly accomplished with fibula osteocutaneous free tissue transfer as an initial reconstructive step. If lower lip elements remain, a large cutaneous paddle can be used to repair oral and mucosal lip defects and replace cutaneous lip, chin, and neck elements. This process can be combined with external advancement and rotation flaps to minimize wound tension and allow for color-matched coverage of a portion of the defect. To reconstruct both internal and external elements, a split double paddle fibula free flap may be used (if robust separate perforators exist) or the central portion of the flap may be de-epithelialized as a more conservative approach. Given the necessity for staged reconstruction, either technique can yield an excellent final result (see **Fig.** 2A–F).

Keys of lower facial reconstruction are to maximize bone-to-bone contact and restore as normal a form as possible, taking care not to underproject the mandible. In cases of severe facial loss, use of a normal sex-matched skull model as a platform to guide reconstructive plate formation serves as a helpful guide. Three-dimensional modeling and reconstruction with plates generated through this technology may provide a more optimal and facile approach in the near future. It is also important to import sufficient skin and soft tissue to both replace lost oral mucosa and prevent fistula (high risk in this population) and to eventually supply sufficient vertical height for the external

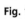

Fig. 1. (*A, B*) An 18 year-old woman with massive injury from a close-range shotgun assault. Defect involves mandible from parasymphysis to contralateral angle, floor of mouth, and ventral tongue, all overlying chin, central neck, and lower lip except orbicualris marginalis and overlying mucosa and extensive upper lip, cheek, left nasal ala, and floor and palate wounds at entry site. (*C*) Postoperative result following split paddle fibula osteocutaneous flap and cheek/neck/lip advancement. (*D*) Interim stage following composite graft for nasal stenosis, upper lip takedown and revision, flap sculpting with 'V' to 'Y' advancement, and scar revision. (*E–G*) Following vestibuloplasty, further external flap excision and lip height increase, placement of dental implants, and fixed maxillomandibular dental prostheses.

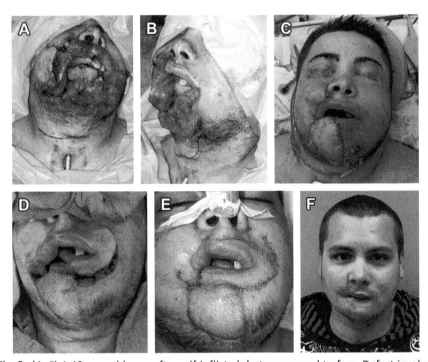

Fig. 2. (*A, B*) A 19-year-old man after self-inflicted shotgun wound to face. Defect involves nearly one-half upper lip, two-thirds lower lip, right commissure, and adjacent cheek, chin, and central neck, as well as mandibular angle to contralateral body and floor of mouth. Palatal splint in place. (*C*) Postoperative after tunneling of remaining lower lip into de-epithelialized fibula skin paddle, native cheek and neck flap advancement, and buccal mucosal turnout for upper lip. (*D, E*) Flap debulking and circumoral myocutaneous lip advancement as second stage and postoperative result. (*F*) Outcome after additional flap sculpting, vestibuloplasty, cervical advancement, and removal of fibula skin paddle.

and internal lower lip. Appropriate lip height is a key to accomplish oral competence and optimize the function of remaining muscular elements.

In cases of mandibular defects combined with loss of total lower lip or greater, remaining lip elements are insufficient to provide for oral competence without unacceptable microstomia. As a result, substantial cutaneous surface area is required to allow for re-creation of vertical lip height; maintaining this skin untethered above the underlying construct is optimal. Given these requirements, reconstruction with 2 separate free flaps may be required (**Fig. 3**A–E). In most patients, radial forearm free flaps are ideal for total lower lip reconstruction given the thinness and pliability of these flaps and the use of palmaris longus tendon for suspension of the lip construct. Anterolateral thigh flaps may be used in thin patients. If patients retain temporalis tendon either unilaterally or bilaterally, palmaris longus or fascia lata suspension to an orthodromic temporalis tendon transfer can provide both oral competence and dynamic lower facial motion (see **Fig. 3**E).

As previously described, subsequent procedures following structural reconstruction are performed following a period of wound maturation. The goal of these procedures is to establish untethered lip height and competence followed by more acceptable aesthetic form. At the same setting, tissue is advanced and color mismatched flap

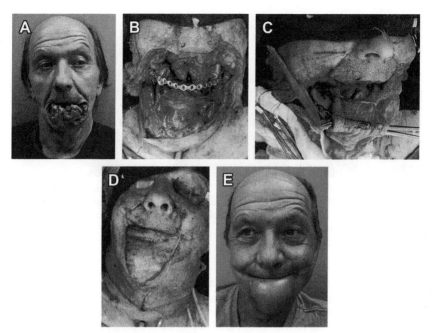

Fig. 3. (*A, B*) Defect of anterior mandible, total lower lip, oral commissures and medial cheeks, chin and central neck, following resection of advanced lip cancer. (*C, D*) Combined fibula osteocutaneous (mandible and floor of mouth) and radial forearm (lower lip and chin) free flaps with bilateral fascia lata suspension to orthodromic temporalis tendon transfers (palmaris longus absent). Postoperative result. (*E*) Dynamic lip competence 1-year postoperatively following radiation therapy.

is excised as possible. Soft tissue bulk in the chin region is typically favorable and preserved and sculpted as overlying skin is removed.

Also, in latter reconstructive stages, circumoral myocutaneous (eg, Karapandzik) or lip switch (eg, Abbe, Estlander) flaps may be used to provide more functional muscular and color-matched lip elements (see **Fig. 2**D, E). Oral vestibuloplasty transferring cutaneous elements from a horizontal floor of the mouth position to a vertical gingivolabial sulcus position provides vertical push on the reconstructed lower lip and allows for thinning of soft tissue over the reconstructed mandible. This critical maneuver both serves as a powerful tool for establishing lip competence and prepares the oral cavity for dental rehabilitation through placement of osseointegrated implants. The latter can be placed at the same setting (**Fig. 4**A–C).

MIDFACE AND PERIORBITAL RECONSTRUCTION

Although isolated massive midface injuries are less commonly encountered, structures may certainly be affected solitarily or in conjunction with severe lower facial injuries; the latter is often the case with self-inflicted blast injuries. Again, initial reconstructive goals are coverage and support of critical structures (eg, eye, palate) and restoration of bony elements to re-establish facial form. The most obvious initial consideration is protection and preservation of the eye. If external lid elements remain, aggressive tarsorraphy during the initial reconstructive stages is often required to accomplish this goal.

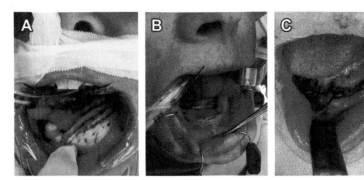

Fig. 4. (*A*, *B*) Oral vestibuloplasty technique. Mature fibula skin paddle divided and de-bulked and then transferred from horizontal to vertical orientation into gingivolabial sulcus to increase lip height. (*C*) Osteointegrated implants are placed, and fibula periostium is left exposed to mucosalize.

Central midface (ie, palatal) trauma may be best managed by a conservative approach such as splinting if elements are severely injured but apparent vascularized soft tissue remains (see **Fig. 2**A). Early intervention in this situation may risk tissue devitalization and further loss. Fistulas that develop may be managed initially or on a long-term basis with dental obturators. As a result, palatal injuries/defects that do not involve key support areas may be best managed with nonsurgical approaches. Reconstruction of central palatal defects at a later stage is often amenable to less invasive minimal access free tissue transfer techniques (**Fig. 5**A–C).

If more lateral midface defects are present and bone elements remain to establish medial and lateral construct stability, midface reconstruction of palatal/orbital/maxillary defects may be amenable to a layered fibula technique.[10] Using this method, fibula and anchored reconstructive plates can allow for preservation of orbital form and eye function even in the setting of defects involving 2 or 3 orbital walls. Keys to this technique include close attention to pedicle geometry and utilization of vascularized soft tissue elements from the free flap to obliterate the maxillary sinus completely and provide complete coverage of orbital plates. The orbital plate is not shaped to re-create absent orbital walls, but rather in the form of a "hammock" to establish orbital volume and globe height appropriately. Careful palpation of the globe and comparison with contralateral eye position serve as the most important guide. If these tenets are used, orbital walls may be reconstructed with titanium mesh plate anchored to skull base, remnant orbital walls, and fibula rim construct alone without additional bone grafts. This technique is well-established in oncologic midface reconstruction with favorable long-term outcomes even in the setting of postoperative radiation therapy (**Fig. 6**A–D).

If large cutaneous and soft tissue defects exist, aggressive replacement and structural suspension is required. Massive lower eyelid and cheek defects may be amenable to layered reconstruction. Aggressive suspension of vascularized fascia lata for inner lamellar reconstruction in conjunction with cutaneous flaps for outer lamellar replacement may provide a viable option for total lower eyelid reconstruction, particularly when upper eyelid elements are not available (**Fig. 7**B). Again, replacement of structure and eye protection is paramount, with contour and color match often left to latter stages (see **Fig. 7**A–C).

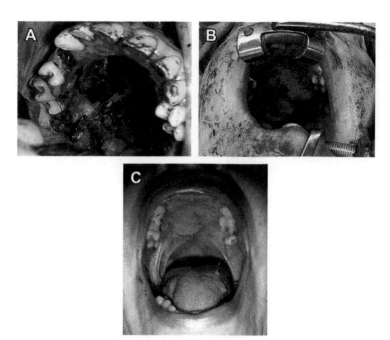

Fig. 5. (*A*) Subtotal hard palate and posterior soft palate and inferior septal defect following tumor resection (note intact alveolus). (*B*) Anterolateral thigh (ALT) fascia lata flap vascualarized via minimal access approach. (*C*) Six-month postoperative result after mucosalization.

NASAL RECONSTRUCTION

In the setting of massive traumatic facial injuries with active forces of contraction and disrupted bony foundations, initial reconstruction of extensive nasal injuries is often best limited to preservation of remaining elements and prevention of further tissue loss and distortion. Following wound maturation and stabilization, approaches for extensive nasal reconstruction mirror traditional techniques used for large defect repair; separate replacement of lining, structure, and cutaneous coverage with a staged approach is required. In this setting, free tissue transfer may be used initially to provide cutaneous coverage of midface and nasal defects. These elements can then be sculpted to provide for lining at later stages. Alternatively, vascularized radial forearm or fascia lata flaps can be used at a later stage for lining replacement. The latter carries the advantage of the ability to provide thin vascularized noncutaneous nasal lining and also provide ample tissue for midface contouring and palatal reconstruction if required (**Fig. 8**A–C).

POSTOPERATIVE CARE AND ANCILLARY PROCEDURES

Postoperative wound care differs from typical reconstructive procedures only in that marginal native tissue breakdown is common. Conservative management with meticulous local wound care and debridement is typically all that is required. Again patient education before reconstruction often mitigates concerns regarding postoperative healing and appearance. In the setting of fistula formation, diversion and conservative management are the most prudent initial course, with repair postponed until tissues mature to the point that further manipulation is tolerated. Often

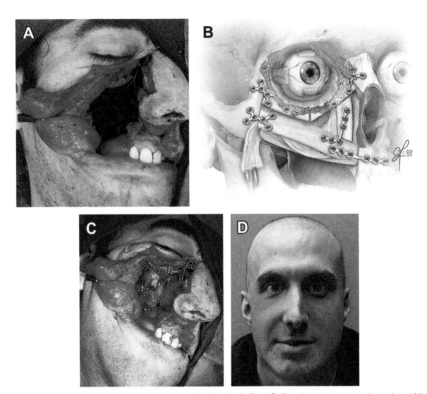

Fig. 6. (*A*) Total maxillectomy and 3-wall orbital defect following tumor extirpation. (*B, C*) Layered fibula technique for orbitomaxillary reconstruction. (*D*) Result at 1 year following postoperative radiation.

with aggressive local wound care small fistulas will close without further surgical intervention.

As stages of reconstruction progress toward more minor revisions, office-based procedures under local anesthesia are often well-tolerated and effective. As the

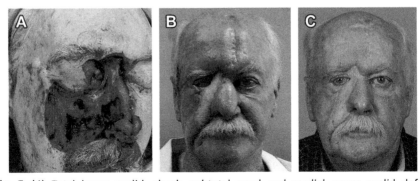

Fig. 7. (*A*) Total lower eyelid, cheek, subtotal nasal and medial upper eyelid defect following tumor resection. (*B*) Postoperative result following ALT fascia lata flap (inner lamella) and radial forearm and cervicofacial flap (outer lamella) reconstruction. (*C*) Preserved eye function 1 year postoperatively following debulking and revision.

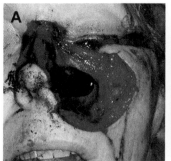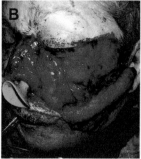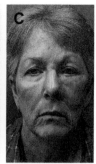

Fig. 8. (*A*) Subtotal nasal, cheek, and maxillary defect. (*B*) Vascularized ALT fascia lata flap for nasal lining and midface contour. (*C*) Result at 1-year postoperatively.

locations of final incisions are determined, scar revision techniques (eg, geometric broken line closures, z-plasty) are performed to minimize visibility and optimize orientation. Further modification techniques (eg, V-beam laser, dermabrasion) may then be used to refine final appearance.

SUMMARY

Free tissue transfer is a critical tool in the management of facial injuries with large composite losses and has led to substantial improvements in reconstructive outcomes. A management philosophy that follows a staged approach to accomplish structural replacement first followed by functional restoration and finally aesthetic form serves as a valuable guide in surgical planning.

REFERENCES

1. Spira M, Hardy SB, Biggs TE, et al. Shotgun injuries of the face. Plast Reconstr Surg 1967;39:449–58.
2. Sherman RT, Parrish RA. Management of shotgun injuries: a review of 152 cases. J Trauma 1963;3:76–86.
3. Vasconez HC, Shockley ME, Luce EA. High energy gunshot wounds to the face. Ann Plast Surg 1996;36:18–25.
4. Gruss JS, Antonyshyn O, Phillips JH. Early definitive bone and soft tissue reconstruction of major gunshot wounds of the face. Plast Reconstr Surg 1991;87:436–50.
5. Finch OR, Oibbell OG. Immediate reconstruction of gunshot wounds to the face. J Trauma 1979;19:965–8.
6. Hidalgo DA. Fibula free flap: a new method of mandible reconstruction. Plast Reconstr Surg 1989;84:71–9.
7. Lukash FN, Sachs SA, Fischma B, et al. Osseointegrated denture in vascularized bone transfer: functional jaw reconstruction. Ann Plast Surg 1987;19:538.
8. Zlotolow IM, Huryn JM, Piro JD, et al. Osseointegrated implants and functional prosthetic rehabilitation in microvascular fibula free flap reconstructed mandibles. Am J Surg 1992;164:677.
9. Urken ML, Buchbinder D, Weinberg H, et al. Primary placement of osseointegrated implants in microvascular mandibular reconstruction. Otolaryngol Head Neck Surg 1989;101:56.
10. Shipchandler T, Waters H, Knott D, et al. Orbitomaxillary reconstruction using the layered fibula osteocutaneous flap. Arch Facial Plas Surg 2012;14(2):110–5.

Index

Note: Page numbers of article titles are in **boldface** type.

A

Alveolar fracture, patterns of, 813
Arch bars, for dental fixation, 817
Auricle, avulsed, after trauma, reconstruction of, **841–855**
　　　tear with nutrient skin pedicle, 842, 843
　　　with existing segment, management of, 842–844
　　defects of, central, reconstruction of, 845
　　　classification of, 844–845
　　　peripheral, reconstruction of, 846–849
　　　prosthetic rehabilitation in, 852–853
　　　secondary reconstruction of, 844–853
　　　subtotal and total, reconstruction of, 849–851, 852
Auricular trauma, surgery in, 842–844

C

Cerebrospinal fluid leak, as complication of cranial base injuries, 750
　　as complication of facial injuries, 742
　　laboratory studies in, 750–751
　　nonsurgical management of, 752
　　surgical management of, 752–755
Computed axial tomography, 720
Computed axial tomography scanners. See *Fan beam CT scanners.*
Condylar fractures, **779–790**
　　closed reduction of, 781
　　complications of, 786–788
　　endoscopic approach to, 785–786, 787
　　intraoral approach to, 784–785
　　outcomes and clinical results of, 789
　　patient positioning for, 780–781
　　pediatric, management considerations in, 798
　　　treatment of, 781
　　postprocedural care in, 788
　　preauricular approach to, 781–782
　　preoperative planning and preparation for, 780
　　procedural approaches in, 781–786
　　rehabilitation and recovery after, 788–789
　　retromandibular approach to, 783–784
　　submandibular/Risdon approach to, 782–783, 784
　　treatment goals and planned outcomes of, 780

Otolaryngol Clin N Am 46 (2013) 915–921
http://dx.doi.org/10.1016/S0030-6665(13)00139-4
0030-6665/13/$ – see front matter © 2013 Elsevier Inc. All rights reserved.

oto.theclinics.com

United States Postal Service

Statement of Ownership, Management, and Circulation
(All Periodicals Publications Except Requestor Publications)

1. Publication Title	2. Publication Number	3. Filing Date
Otolaryngologic Clinics of North America	4 6 6 - 5 5 5 0	9/14/13

4. Issue Frequency	5. Number of Issues Published Annually	6. Annual Subscription Price
Feb, Apr, Jun, Aug, Oct, Dec	6	$348.00

7. Complete Mailing Address of Known Office of Publication (Not printer) (Street, city, county, state, and ZIP+4®)

Elsevier Inc.
360 Park Avenue South
New York, NY 10010-1710

Contact Person: Stephen R. Bushing
Telephone (Include area code): 215-239-3688

8. Complete Mailing Address of Headquarters or General Business Office of Publisher (Not printer)

Elsevier Inc., 360 Park Avenue South, New York, NY 10010-1710

9. Full Names and Complete Mailing Addresses of Publisher, Editor, and Managing Editor (Do not leave blank)

Publisher (Name and complete mailing address)

Linda Belfus, Elsevier, Inc., 1600 John F. Kennedy Blvd. Suite 1800, Philadelphia, PA 19103-2899

Editor (Name and complete mailing address)

Joanne Husovski, Elsevier, Inc., 1600 John F. Kennedy Blvd. Suite 1800, Philadelphia, PA 19103-2899

Managing Editor (Name and complete mailing address)

Adrianne Brigido, Elsevier, Inc., 1600 John F. Kennedy Blvd. Suite 1800, Philadelphia, PA 19103-2899

10. Owner (Do not leave blank. If the publication is owned by a corporation, give the name and address of the corporation immediately followed by the names and addresses of all stockholders owning or holding 1 percent or more of the total amount of stock. If not owned by a corporation, give the names and addresses of the individual owners. If owned by a partnership or other unincorporated firm, give its name and address as well as those of each individual owner. If the publication is published by a nonprofit organization, give its name and address.)

Full Name	Complete Mailing Address
Wholly owned subsidiary of	1600 John F. Kennedy Blvd., Ste. 1800
Reed/Elsevier, US holdings	Philadelphia, PA 19103-2899

11. Known Bondholders, Mortgagees, and Other Security Holders Owning or Holding 1 Percent or More of Total Amount of Bonds, Mortgages, or Other Securities. If none, check box ☐ None

Full Name	Complete Mailing Address
N/A	

12. Tax Status (For completion by nonprofit organizations authorized to mail at nonprofit rates) (Check one)
The purpose, function, and nonprofit status of this organization and the exempt status for federal income tax purposes:
☐ Has Not Changed During Preceding 12 Months
☐ Has Changed During Preceding 12 Months (Publisher must submit explanation of change with this statement)

PS Form 3526, September 2007 (Page 1 of 3 (Instructions Page 3)) PSN 7530-01-000-9931 PRIVACY NOTICE: See our Privacy policy in www.usps.com

---

13. Publication Title	14. Issue Date for Circulation Data Below
Otolaryngologic Clinics of North America	June 2013

15. Extent and Nature of Circulation		Average No. Copies Each Issue During Preceding 12 Months	No. Copies of Single Issue Published Nearest to Filing Date
a. Total Number of Copies (Net press run)		1229	1174
b. Paid Circulation (By Mail and Outside the Mail)	(1) Mailed Outside-County Paid Subscriptions Stated on PS Form 3541. (Include paid distribution above nominal rate, advertiser's proof copies, and exchange copies)	549	494
	(2) Mailed In-County Paid Subscriptions Stated on PS Form 3541 (Include paid distribution above nominal rate, advertiser's proof copies, and exchange copies)		
	(3) Paid Distribution Outside the Mails Including Sales Through Dealers and Carriers, Street Vendors, Counter Sales, and Other Paid Distribution Outside USPS®	379	338
	(4) Paid Distribution by Other Classes Mailed Through the USPS (e.g. First-Class Mail®)		
c. Total Paid Distribution (Sum of 15b (1), (2), (3), and (4))		928	832
d. Free or Nominal Rate Distribution (By Mail and Outside the Mail)	(1) Free or Nominal Rate Outside-County Copies Included on PS Form 3541	74	26
	(2) Free or Nominal Rate In-County Copies Included on PS Form 3541		
	(3) Free or Nominal Rate Copies Mailed at Other Classes Through the USPS (e.g. First-Class Mail)		
	(4) Free or Nominal Rate Distribution Outside the Mail (Carriers or other means)		
e. Total Free or Nominal Rate Distribution (Sum of 15d (1), (2), (3) and (4))		74	26
f. Total Distribution (Sum of 15c and 15e)		1002	858
g. Copies not Distributed (See instructions to publishers #4 (page #3))		227	316
h. Total (Sum of 15f and g)		1229	1174
i. Percent Paid (15c divided by 15f times 100)		92.61%	96.97%

16. Publication of Statement of Ownership
☐ If the publication is a general publication, publication of this statement is required. Will be printed in the December 2013 issue of this publication. ☐ Publication not required

17. Signature and Title of Editor, Publisher, Business Manager, or Owner

Stephen R. Bushing — Inventory/Distribution Coordinator   Date September 14, 2013

I certify that all information furnished on this form is true and complete. I understand that anyone who furnishes false or misleading information on this form or who omits material or information requested on the form may be subject to criminal sanctions (including fines and imprisonment) and/or civil sanctions (including civil penalties).

PS Form 3526, September 2007 (Page 2 of 3)

Moving?

Make sure your subscription moves with you!

To notify us of your new address, find your **Clinics Account Number** (located on your mailing label above your name), and contact customer service at:

Email: journalscustomerservice-usa@elsevier.com

800-654-2452 (subscribers in the U.S. & Canada)
314-447-8871 (subscribers outside of the U.S. & Canada)

Fax number: 314-447-8029

Elsevier Health Sciences Division
Subscription Customer Service
3251 Riverport Lane
Maryland Heights, MO 63043

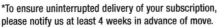

*To ensure uninterrupted delivery of your subscription, please notify us at least 4 weeks in advance of move.

Printed and bound by CPI Group (UK) Ltd, Croydon, CR0 4YY

03/10/2024

01040492-0004